D1569498

Life After
DEAF

Life After
DEAF

*my misadventures
in hearing loss and recovery*

NOEL HOLSTON

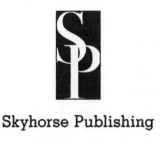

Skyhorse Publishing

Skyhorse Publishing books may be purchased in bulk at special discounts for
sales promotion, corporate gifts, fund-raising, or educational purposes. Special
editions can also be created to specifications. For details, contact the Special
Sales Department, Skyhorse Publishing, 307 West 36th Street, 11th Floor, New
York, NY 10018 or info@skyhorsepublishing.com.

Skyhorse® and Skyhorse Publishing® are registered trademarks of Skyhorse
Publishing, Inc.®, a Delaware corporation.

Visit our website at www.skyhorsepublishing.com.

10 9 8 7 6 5 4 3 2

Library of Congress Cataloging-in-Publication Data is available on file.

Cover design by Paul Qualcom
Cover image credit: Getty Images

Print ISBN: 978-1-5107-4687-9
Ebook ISBN: 978-1-5107-4688-6

Printed in the United States of America

For Marty, my spark

Table of Contents

Author's Note

This is a book about how going deaf changed my life, my identity, my marriage, my relationship with the world. It's a chronicle of what I've done to cope, what I've learned about hearing loss and communication, and what it might be like for you or someone in your life. An estimated 40 million American are deaf or hearing impaired. Our numbers grow every day.

... and therefore never send to know for whom
the bell tolls; it tolls for thee.
—John Donne

Bell? What bell?
—Noel Holston

Introduction

Usually, the purpose of an introduction is to do precisely that: introduce the reader to a book's subject, tone, and author, as a place setter for what is to follow. But already, before arriving to this point, the reader has been handed significant hints from the author himself.

The book's very title, *Life After Deaf,* is a giveaway tell that Noel Holston not only is not above the occasional puns, but revels and wallows in wordplay. The author's note, placed before these pages, clearly establishes the book's approach to the subject of being hearing impaired, a focus at once contextually wide and personally specific. By telling his own story so honestly, Noel manages to shed light on scores of millions of others. And the third piece of evidence supplied by the author in the pages before this intro, the overleaf, is the capper: He betrays his love of literature and popular culture by quoting John Donne, then follows it with his own unexpected, wry rejoinder. As I read the galleys for this book, that hilarious one-two punch truly made me laugh out loud—and the book itself hadn't even started yet. Those early clues, taken together, are ample early evidence of what you can expect to experience throughout *Life After Deaf:* an uncommon combination of incisive intelligence and playful humor.

Long before Noel Holston finally decided to write his memoir and become an author, he toiled, as I did and still do, in the field of TV criticism. As such, he was one of the very best writers on the beat, and also one of the best reporters and analysts. Those are three distinctly different skills, and all three are the secret weapons he employs when turning his focus inward. Because of his background as a reporter, Noel does the necessary research to know what he's talking about, asks all the right questions, and pays attention to the actions and reactions of those around him. He's honest enough to describe what he's feeling, and hearing or not hearing, every step of the way, so he takes you with him from start to finish. And he's such a good writer that he's always making references and observations that help ground his story and make it relatable, while trusting that, especially in writing a memoir, honesty is the best policy. As a result, *Life After Deaf* is a bravely unfiltered and wide-ranging voyage, with Noel as a charming tour guide—taking you not only deep inside his ear canal, but deep inside his marriage and his mind, as well.

By telling his own story so personally, and so personably, Noel has written something here that is more than just informative or inspirational—though it's both of those, big-time. *Life After Deaf,* as I read it, also is a love letter. He doesn't omit or neglect the feelings of his wife and family and freely acknowledges that, as with anyone suffering through any malady or tragedy, those burdens are seldom carried alone. By including those around him in his story, even when observing how much his behavior is irritating them, the tale he's telling is more relatable, more empathetic, and ultimately more real.

This book can be read as a primer: what to expect, and perhaps what to avoid, when noticing that your auditory senses are beginning to wane significantly. And as a memoir, telling the story of a writer who finds ways to adapt as both his journalistic career and his hearing skills shift through the years. But please don't underestimate the power of Noel's storytelling, and his love of music and pop culture, laced through every page of this narrative. It's what ultimately makes this very serious memoir so funny and joyful. References come from all over and pop up at unexpected times, yet always stick their landings, whether he's comparing a cockeyed mechanics of the human ear to a Rube Goldberg contraption or making apt references to the Marvel comic superhero Daredevil or David Seville's novelty hit "Witch Doctor." And I'm sorry—but when a retirement-age white man with hearing problems refers to himself as "Mos Deaf," he deserves, if not demands, to be heard.

And hearing, after all, is at the center of Noel's story. Turn the page and experience it for yourself...

—David Bianculli, *Fresh Air* TV Critic
and Rowan University professor of TV Studies

Chapter 1
Monkey Business

Our bedroom was chilly when I slid out of bed and stumbled into the bathroom to relieve myself. It was the beginning of my winter daybreak ritual: Get up. Relieve. Wash hands. Clomp downstairs. Turn up thermostat. Turn on coffee maker. Feed cats.

But as I stood over the toilet in the nightlight's blue glow, I heard no splash. "Hmm," I murmured to myself.

The hmm was inaudible, too. I stepped over to the sink and turned the handle. The water I saw rushing from the faucet was a silent stream. "Hmm," I murmured again.

I surveyed my face in the medicine cabinet mirror. I watched my left hand as I reached up and rubbed my left ear. The sound it made was faint, distant, and dull as cotton. I rubbed my right ear with my right hand. Nothing. Nothing at all.

I shuffled back to bed and lay down next to my wife, eyes fixed on the ceiling. I woke Marty, not meaning to, with what I would have sworn was whispering. I was mouthing words—names, numbers, snippets of songs—hoping to find a tone, a pitch, that would register as sound. She told me later that her first sleepy thought when my mumbling woke her was that I had suffered a stroke.

"Honey, what's wrong?" she asked. Her face loomed over me like a pale moon. I responded to her worried look, not her words.

"Your lips are moving," I said, "but there's no sound."

"Nothing?" she said.

I shook my head.

She came around to my side of the bed and switched on the brass lamp on my nightstand. She motioned for me to sit up and then pushed a folded pillow behind me. Marty is medically knowledgeable. One of the many day jobs she's worked in her life as a singer, songwriter, and musician is certified nurse's attendant. She wanted to look me over and assess whether we needed to race to the nearest emergency room.

She plucked a tissue from the box on our bookcase headboard. "Blow your nose," she said, miming the gesture.

I blew, careful not to push too hard, and then again, harder. She gave me a how-now look. I shook my head and shrugged my befuddlement.

She put her face up close to my left ear. I could faintly detect the word "sleep." I lay back down on my side. She switched off the light and crawled back into bed with me.

Though she was spooned against my back, I was alone in my thoughts. I took stock. My left ear had faded over a period of half a dozen years, starting in the mid-1990s. I'd had a series of hearing aids. My good ear, the right, had been getting weaker, though gradually. I had composed a sort of prose poem (see *Dropping the Needle*, page 197) a few days earlier. It extolled my ability to summon familiar music from memory. I had planned to perform it later in the week at Word of Mouth, a monthly poetry and spoken-word jam at a downtown bar in Athens, Georgia, where we live. It was a knack that I had presumed would come in handy in the event my hearing ever got really, really bad. But I had never expected a loss so sudden, so dramatic. I had been fending off a mild cold and was sniffling a bit, but surely that couldn't be the instigation for what seemed close to a total collapse.

The night before, March 3, 2010, I had gone to bed able to hear all manner of everyday sounds and comprehend conversation easily with a little amplification. Yet here I was on the morning of March 4 so auditorily challenged I could only faintly detect the sound of my own voice in my head.

I lay there cuddled up to Marty trying to will myself unconscious, hoping I could indeed sleep it off. The prospect of a silent or near-silent existence didn't scare me to death—I understood, intellectually at least, that there are millions of people who live and work and play without any hearing at all. I only felt a wave of sadness. I had never been good with quiet. I was raised in a household in which there was almost always a record player or a radio going, sometimes more than one. I had spent sixty years in a sonic marinade.

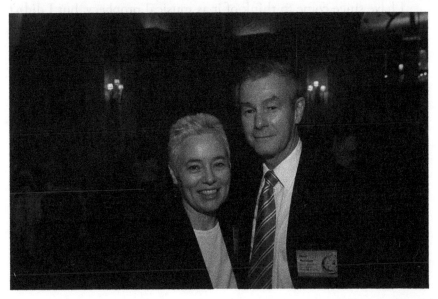

Courtesy of Peabody Awards

My thoughts floated to music, which I love as much if not more than conversation. In recent weeks, I had been driving around with a boom box in the front seat of my old Mazda because, for some reason, its tone worked better with my weakened ears than the in-dash stereo. I had been playing a CD that had been a promotional gimme for an Elvis Presley retrospective that his ex-wife, Priscilla, had produced for television. For many years I had critiqued TV programming for a living. Friends and newspaper colleagues never got tired of predicting that my brain was going to turn to mush or that I would go blind. Maybe they were onto something.

The CD included rare alternative recordings of a few Elvis hits and some oddball studio outtakes. The last music I had heard on March 3 was Elvis and some of his pals goofing on an old Chuck Berry song, "Too Much Monkey Business," a madcap, tongue-twisting litany of hassles, hoops, indignities, and idiocies the hero has had to duckwalk his way around and through.

I have since come to think of it as musical prophecy, but I didn't realize that morning just how apt it would be, a theme song for my adventures in hearing impairment, for the comedy of errors to come. Monkey business indeed.

Chapter 2

Doctor, Doctor

M arty shook me awake an hour later. I was still hearing only the sounds of silence. It was strange, disorienting, and worrisome, but I resisted the urge to panic. Once, years earlier, my hearing nosedived during a flight from a press event in New York City back to Florida, where I wrote for a daily newspaper, the *Orlando Sentinel*. I suddenly couldn't hear the passenger seated next to me. I couldn't hear myself swallow. Flight attendants' faces bobbed above me, their lips moving silently. It was surreal and alarming. But it was caused by head-cold congestion and cabin-pressure change. It cleared up by the time I got to baggage claim. Maybe this was just something similar. Maybe I just had waxy yellow build-up.

Not knowing what else to do, I got up and had breakfast with Marty. I did my usual stretch routine, including rolling back and throwing my legs over my head. I took a long, hot shower and tugged on my earlobes as Marty had shown me, hoping to clear my Eustachian tubes. No dice.

Marty, meanwhile, attempted to reach Dr. Ronald Leif Steenerson, a highly regarded otologist in Atlanta. I had seen him the previous fall in hopes that he could help me with tinnitus— ringing in my ears. He had diagnosed my problem as excess fluid in my inner ears. He prescribed a mild diuretic and told me to hide the saltshaker and do my best to resist the temptations of bacon and pepperoni. Steenerson was out of the country on vacation when Marty phoned his office.

I got dressed and went to my office at the University of Georgia's journalism school. I'm a notoriously dutiful worker bee. Marty never lets me forget the time when we were living in Minneapolis and she phoned me at the newspaper, the *Star Tribune*, and told me she'd fallen on a flight of stairs at the theater where she worked. She was worried her leg might be broken. She says that I said, "Oh, that's terrible, honey, but I'm on deadline. Can someone else take you to the ER? I'll get there as soon as I turn my column in!" Her memory is probably accurate.

Driving toward the university, it was surreal not being able to tell if my car was running except by looking at the dashboard lights and stranger still to have to tell my colleagues by email to pass me notes if they wanted to converse with me.

As the day wore on, however, I realized I was hearing a bit more. I emailed Marty and told her it appeared she had been right, that getting up and moving around had shaken the mucous or the crud or whatever out of my head. We laughed about our overreaction when I came home. For dinner we had her special chicken soup, freshly made and hopped up with spices, extra garlic, and fresh ginger. Its therapeutic and decongestant properties are legendary in our household, and she thought it would not only cure my sniffles, but reinvigorate my sinuses and ears.

After eating a big bowl and inhaling the redolent steam, I sat down with her to watch an evening newscast. Halfway through, I reached across the sofa and tapped her on the knee. "Honey," I said quietly. "It's gone again. I can't hear a thing."

Our hope of letting my ear problem work itself out dashed, Marty got on the phone to my younger brother, Tim. He was then an audiology professor at the University of South Alabama in Mobile and the coordinator of its hearing clinic. Tim was very concerned.

He told Marty that sudden, severe hearing loss ideally needs to be treated within a week of its onset if there's going to be much chance of restoration. The window for action is small.

"Don't put this off," he said. "He needs to see a doctor tomorrow."

We slept fitfully, annoyed with ourselves. First thing the next morning, Marty found the phone number for an ear, nose, and throat specialist in Athens. She made a call and got me a midday appointment with a doctor who, as it turned out, looked as though he could be singing lead in a Kenny Rogers tribute band. Learning that Marty was a singer, he started talking to her about his love of country music. It aggravated me that he couldn't seem to comprehend how little of what he said I could understand. One would think an ear doctor would have a better appreciation of deafness, but no. He blabbed on and on, seemingly oblivious to the fact that, to me, he was a TV talking head and the mute button was on. Marty appraised him of my cold and slight congestion, but he prescribed no drug, no antibiotic, just patience—wait and see and it'll probably bounce back.

We weren't happy with his plan of inaction, but there was no other ENT practice nearby that was in my Blue Cross Blue Shield of Georgia insurance network, and we were unfamiliar with Atlanta, an hour-and-a-half drive away. We grudgingly took Kenny's advice. We gambled and waited for Dr. Steenerson to return from his trip. By the time I did get to see him, on March 15, or ten days later, my window apparently had slammed shut.

Steenerson is a tall, bald man with military bearing. He's a serious sport fisherman who has marlins hanging on the walls of his waiting room. Fishing and hunting magazines share the racks with *Vanity Fair* and *Elle*. He has a cabin in Montana. We had been cautioned before my first appointment with him about his lack of bedside manner, and he had not disappointed. He was only slightly warmer than the big fish on his walls. Marty is playful and elfin, part Peter Pan, part Cyndi Lauper. She has been known to charm rocks. So she was determined to establish a human connection with Steenerson this time around.

"Nice boots," she said, nodding toward his cowboy footwear.

"What?" he said, looking annoyed to be interrupted.

"Nice boots," she repeated. "I grew up in Nebraska. I know nice boots when I see 'em."

He cocked a disapproving fuzzy eyebrow at her. He grunted and went back to looking in my ear with an otoscope.

We came to understand that as gruff and cranky as he sometimes seemed, what we were experiencing was actually his extreme focus as he processed what he saw and heard from his patient. He's a good, generous fellow, beloved by his staff.

After conducting a physical examination of my right ear, Steenerson had one of the audiologists on his staff put me in a sound-proof testing booth to determine which tones I could hear and which words, if any, I could comprehend. I dutifully punched a button when I detected faint beeps in my headphones and then attempted to repeat simple words the audiologist read. Studying the pitiful results, Steenerson explained that I had experienced a sensorineural loss. The cilia—the microscopic hairs in my inner ear that wave in the breezes of sound like a wheat field or a kelp forest—had been knocked over and flattened. They had fallen and couldn't get up.

Marty translated what I couldn't understand, either speaking directly to my face with exaggerated mouth movements or writing on a note pad.

I asked if he could tell what had caused the sudden drop-off. Steenerson told us it could be viral, allergenic, a reaction to medication, or the result of a blow to the head.

I couldn't remember the last time I had been ill with anything worse than indigestion or a middling cold. I was ridiculously healthy. My only allergy is to penicillin and thus bread mold, which makes me break out in hives and blows up my lips and tongue, but

I hadn't had a bad-muffin episode in ages. The only medication I was taking daily was a multivitamin and occasional niacin tablet for my tinnitus. As for blows to the head, there was that time I hit loose gravel on my bike on the way to a Cub Scout meeting, fell headlong onto the pavement, and spent half a day out cold. There were the innumerable times I had been battered by bad-hop baseballs. But those were childhood lumps. I hadn't been hit by anybody or anything as an adult since, well, since I accidentally offended a drunk at a bar while I was living on Long Island, New York, and writing for *Newsday*. But even that sucker punch to the head was a good five years before my ears went kaput.

Steenerson arranged for some tests, including an MRI. That would be standard procedure anyway, but there was also a red-flag medical history matter: my father developed a malignant brain tumor and died at the age of forty-seven, when I was still a teenager. I was now sixty-two.

If you've never had an MRI, it's an acronym for magnetic resonance imaging. Instructed to hold deadly still, the patient is slid into a sort of fiberglass and metal womb and bombarded with magnetic impulses that generate computer images of bone and tissue. It looks like something Dr. McCoy would use to diagnose ailing crew members on the Starship Enterprise. While it scans you, it makes creaking, whirring, thumping noises that sound like the warm-up of a rhythmically challenged polka band. The magnetism is so strong, neither patient nor technician can be in the same room with the machine while wearing a watch. If you happen to have a steel plate in your skull or a pin in your ankle, forget it. It will glom onto you as if it were a refrigerator and you were a magnet encased in a little plastic butterfly. Some people find the prospect of getting scanned about as appealing as being sealed in a coffin. But I didn't mind. I just closed my eyes and imagined I was lying on a beach. To my barely functioning left ear, the MRI's rattle and clunk sounded vaguely like lapping waves.

The scan found nothing amiss, so it was back to guessing the cause. Dr. Steenerson said it actually didn't make much difference as far as treatment was concerned. Whatever the cause, the effect was what he had to treat. And there were only so many options available to him.

I breathed a secret sigh of relief that he hadn't told me loud music was the culprit. The thought had crossed my mind more than once. What if I was like the longtime smoker who had gambled that lung cancer or emphysema only happened to other people? What if I was like the guy who never met a chocolate bar or a lemon drop he didn't like and who one fine morning gets a diabetes diagnosis? What if the music I loved so much and was already missing terribly was in fact a cause? I had told myself that I hadn't abused my ears nearly as much as many guys my age. I was never one to live with headphones on. I had stopped going to mega-amped concerts years earlier. My brother the audiologist, who knows better, was far more likely to ride around in a sealed automobile with Joe Bonamassa ripping scorching blues licks at top volume. And he could still hear.

I was thrilled that Dr. Steenerson let me off the hook. Neither I nor U2 was to blame. It was a mystery.

Chapter 3

Whispers in Bedlam

D r. Steenerson's first line of attack was to put me on a daily steroid dosage. With luck, he believed, it might still snap my fallen cilia to attention.

The first couple of days I was on Prednisone, nothing much changed. I experienced slightly improved hearing in my right ear for two or three hours after I woke up, but it faded in the afternoon, and, by night, I couldn't understand Marty's words from a foot away, much less the narration of a newscaster on television.

Then came a personal Big Bang. On the third day of Prednisone, the hair cells in my cochlea rose from the dead. I had driven to the Athens YMCA, where we had a membership, to work out. After riding a stationary bike for twenty minutes to get my heart pumping, stretching, and then lifting some weights, I started down the hall from the fitness area to the locker room. I was jolted by what seemed like surround sound at a movie theater. It was as if a stereo system had just been turned on. Loud. I heard a wonderful squealing melee of children playing in the Y's several gyms. I could detect conversations among people walking ten to fifteen feet ahead of me. I hadn't heard so much sound in years.

Outside in the parking lot, I could hear birds and the swoosh and rumble of cars and trucks passing on Hawthorne Avenue. When I started my car, it wasn't just the faint, dull groan to which I had become accustomed. I heard the key turn in the ignition. I heard the engine crackle to life and roar. I heard the squeak of a fan belt and the rattle of my key chain clacking against the dashboard as I drove away.

I turned on the radio, preset to WUGA, the University of Georgia radio station. National Public Radio's Renée Montagne was reading a news report. I could understand her. It was as though she were in the passenger's seat next to me. "Hello, Renée!" I shouted.

At an intersection a block away, I stopped for the red light. A car pulled up in the turn lane on my left. My window was open, and so were theirs. I could hear the two guys in the car talking. I turned my radio down. The guys were discussing where they were going to go for a beer. I could make out some of what they were saying over the rock music playing in *their* car. It sounded familiar. I concentrated hard. I recognized the cadence. Yes! Allman Brothers' "Rambling Man." It felt as though my whole body had been zapped with a rejuvenating ray. I felt so alive. I wanted to cry. I wanted to dance.

As I drove on toward home, a distant memory popped into my head. A title: "Whispers in Bedlam." It's an Irwin Shaw short story that I had read in *Playboy* decades earlier. I really did buy it for the articles. Mostly.

Shaw's story is about a journeyman National Football League defensive player who undergoes surgery to repair a hearing problem and ends up with ears like Superman's. He can overhear the opposing team's offensive huddles, and his seemingly supernatural ability to anticipate plays makes him a sudden sensation.

I didn't feel like an all-star, but I felt exhilarated. I could hear with a precision I could never remember having. I had what Marty calls "country ears"—hearing like a hunter, like a deer, like a bobcat.

I couldn't wait to get home to listen to her. We sat on the love seat in our TV nook and talked and talked and talked. It was exhausting. It was heaven.

That night, we watched the new episode of *Lost* on ABC. I didn't turn on the wireless headphone apparatus that my stepdaughter, Downie, had bought for me so I wouldn't have to turn the TV volume up so loud for everyone else. I understood what the characters were saying. I heard them. Every word.

The miracle was short-lived.

The next morning when I awakened, my speech comprehension was weaker. It picked up after I had my black coffee, granola, and Prednisone tablets, but it didn't reach the giddy, preternatural level of the previous day. By week's end, I was back to having a slight improvement starting around midmorning and then inevitably segueing into life as silent movie by midafternoon.

I also began to recognize another manifestation of hearing loss. Even when it was suspected that the cause of my tinnitus was Meniere's disease, I had not suffered the dizziness and loss of balance that often accompanies that syndrome. I remained lucky on that count. What was impaired, however, was my ability to use my hearing to gauge my physical place in the world.

We don't think of ourselves as having an internal sounding system—sonar, like bats or whales. We hear no "ping, ping" like the crew of a deep-diving submarine. Yet we do use our hearing, in concert with our vision, to continuously monitor our spatial relationship to people and things. Our brains make ongoing, unconscious calculations from all our sensory input to keep us from wheeling around suddenly and whacking a stranger in the face when we're waiting in line to purchase tickets to a movie or to buy our groceries. We hear faint echoes that help us know how low to duck our heads when we climb into a car. Hearing helps us gauge where we end and the rest of the world begins.

At my most deaf, I banged my head getting in and out my car and cracked my noggin on the underside of kitchen cabinet doors I forgot I had opened. I had to start making a conscious effort to notice spatial relationships. It was either that or buy a football helmet.

* * *

The last week of that March was torture. For three decades, I had made my living covering arts and entertainment, primarily television, for a succession of newspapers. After I left *Newsday* in the fall of 2005 and relocated to Athens, I lucked into the offer of a part-time job doing public relations for the University of Georgia-based George Foster Peabody Awards, which is akin to a Pulitzer Prize for TV and radio and a *Good Housekeeping* seal of approval.

My job at the Peabodys included writing press releases and articles for our website and staging and promoting events—screenings of winning programs and speaking engagements by winners on the University campus. But the crucial chore was to take notes during the annual judging process and write the winners-announcement news bulletin and the descriptive "citations" that appear in the souvenir program of the ceremony we staged every spring in New York. The citations are intended to reflect the deliberations of the Peabody board.

The judges winnow more than a thousand entries down to a list of about thirty winners. It takes them four days. Four 9 a.m. to 6 p.m. (sometimes 7 or 8 p.m.) days of near-constant chatter. Trying to catch a quotable phrase here and there requires intense, constant concentration.

The process was challenging for me even when my hearing was still pretty good. Fifteen board members, the Peabody director, and assorted staffers sit at or around a long table in a narrow, high-ceiling room watching clips from TV and radio programs entered in the competition. Board members report on shows they've been assigned to view ahead of convening in Athens and recommend submissions they deem worthy of further evaluation. And they argue. Oh, how they argue. As they tout personal favorite programs and express misgivings about others, the sessions begin to resemble an intense scene from the famous jury-trial movie, *12 Angry Men*. People talk over one another, playing verbal King of the Hill. A tossed-off quip I miss cracks up the room, the big laugh eclipsing any and all ripostes. Some Peabody jurors are quiet-voiced, "low talkers" in *Seinfeld* parlance. Some judges mumble. No matter whom I sit next to, some panelists at the table are out of my range. I would sometimes find myself as badly overmatched as I would be playing tennis with one of the Williams sisters. Well, almost.

My solution this time, with my steroid-treated hearing weaker and unpredictable, was to flit around the edges of the table, constantly repositioning myself for optimum proximity to whoever was speaking. I felt like a human pinball, literally bouncing off the walls.

Ultimately, there were too few understandable words and too much sound. Group laughter was a blitzkrieg for my sickly ears, an auditory assault. It was exhausting, and the impact lingered. In the quiet of my car driving home, my ears would ring as though I had been at a shooting range all day without any protective eargear. The board members arrived at their unanimous winners list Sunday morning, April 4, said their farewells, and headed to Atlanta to catch planes home to places as far flung as Ann Arbor and Hong Kong. I had never been so happy to see them leave. I composed the citations over the next two days in my office with the door shut.

* * *

What would prove to be one of my most embarrassing and humbling incidents of my near-deaf days happened in mid-April. I got to the back door of the Peabody Awards offices one workday morning and realized I didn't have my key. I hiked around to the front of the building, got the receptionist to let me in, put my backpack and a bag of DVDs on a chair in the lobby, and headed back up the long, steep hill to the university ramp where I park.

I climbed the stairs to the third floor, and there was my Mazda. Running. I could see a light stream of exhaust fumes coming out the tailpipe. I ran to the car and pulled on the front door handle. Locked. I barked a long string of expletives I could not hear. I had apparently gotten distracted when I had gotten out of the car. Not being able to hear the warning beeper, let alone the engine, I had instinctively flipped the lock and walked away.

I'm a longtime AAA member, but I couldn't call for assistance. Couldn't hear. Couldn't text them, either. AAA doesn't do texting. I texted Marty, but she didn't reply. I remembered she had gone to a medical appointment.

I walked back down the hill to the Peabodys, sheepishly told a colleague what had happened, and asked if she could drive me to my house to get my spare keys. We drove, of course, in silence.

I had no door key, either, but there was a possibility. Our house, like so many houses in hilly Athens, is built on an incline. The front of the house rests on solid ground, the back on stilts, fifteen feet high. We have a deck off the back of the house, a deck for which there are no stairs. There is a sliding glass door to the deck. We seldom lock it. I asked my colleague to wait. I dragged a garbage can alongside a corner post of the deck, turned the receptacle over, and climbed on top of it. From there, I was able to reach a crossbeam. I pulled myself up and began to shimmy up toward the railing. It was like being a kid on a jungle gym—the maneuver, not me. I found myself using muscles and contorting my body in ways it hadn't been contorted in decades. I would be feeling it for days.

I managed to drag myself up and over the railing. The sliding door wasn't locked, thank God. I found the spare keys, changed clothes—my khakis and shirt were dirty from the climb—and zipped out the door to my colleague's car. Ten minutes later, she dropped me off by the parking ramp. I unlocked my car and turned it off. Then I restarted it briefly so I could look at the fuel gauge. I had burned about a quarter tank. I took some comfort in knowing I was still getting pretty decent mileage.

* * *

In late April, on Dr. Steenerson's referral, I went to see an Atlanta rheumatologist, Dr. Alan B. Fishman. With the oral steroid failing to have permanent impact, Steenerson speculated that my problem might be autoimmune. Fishman was personable, warm even, and clearly knew his stuff. And he wasn't prone to feel-good promises. He prescribed a regimen of methotrexate, a drug developed to treat certain types of lung, breast, and skin cancer but also prescribed at times to treat rheumatoid arthritis and other autoimmune illnesses like lupus and Crohn's disease. The idea behind it is that the immune system has erroneously identified a destructive agent in the ear and is, in effect, attacking the ear itself.

Methotrexate is serious medication. Dr. Fishman initially prescribed a low dosage, three 2.5 mg tablets per week, just to make sure it didn't curdle my stomach. Once I embarked on the stronger, daily dosage ten days later, I had to get a blood test once a week to make sure it wasn't damaging my liver or kidneys. After a few weeks, I was such a familiar figure at LabCorp, a testing facility in Athens, that the staff hailed my entrances—well, they waved— as though I were Norm Peterson, the genial barfly in the sitcom *Cheers*, sauntering toward his stool. I was on a first-name basis with three phlebotomists.

I was doing my best not to give up on getting out and about. In late April, Marty was the warm-up act for singer-songwriter Loudon Wainwright III at The Melting Point, an Athens music club. She'd opened for him in the past when we lived in Minneapolis and on Long Island. As a thank-you at the Athens show, she surprised him with her rendition of "Kick in the Head," his bitterly funny song about being cuckolded by a friend. Wainwright himself, notoriously prickly, was in unusually generous form, even honoring a request late in his show for his biggest hit, the novelty tune "Dead Skunk." The Melting Point sound system was so loud I actually recognized what he was singing from the cadence—well, that and the fact it's a banjo tune. Good visual cue. And since I knew the song well, I could fill in words I couldn't understand. But when friends who joined us at our table tried to talk to me during the breaks, I had to pull my trusty stenographer's pad from my bag and pass it around. I went home thinking of the night as a draw.

In mid-May, Marty and I flew to New York for the Peabody Awards ceremony. The director insisted I go, though not in a taskmaster sense. It was more a reward. My main work, promoting the event and writing winners' citations and copy for the souvenir program, was done well before I got on a plane. On ceremony day, my main function is shmoozing the press. I found I could glad-hand without hearing and fake my way through small talk. The reporters in attendance were so preoccupied they scarcely noticed I was mainly nodding and smiling.

Honorees at the ceremony in the Waldorf-Astoria grand ballroom included CNN's exhaustive coverage of the previous year's Gulf of Mexico oil spill, *The Good Wife*, a *Washington Post* website series about traumatic brain injuries, and a dazzling science series, *Wonders of the Solar System*. The Peabody show was, as always, megaloud, the volume pumped up to ensure no one in the cavernous hall could not hear. Even I could make out many of the words spoken from the podium.

As the representatives of thirty-plus winning programs took their turns coming on stage and making their acceptance speeches, it crossed my mind that just two years earlier, the Peabodys had honored *Hear and Now,* a bittersweet documentary by a woman whose parents, lifelong deaf, decided to undergo cochlear implant surgery and had distinctly different reactions to their rendezvous with sound. The wife was thrilled to hear sound for the first time in her life, but her husband not so much, and it had caused a rift. I had made a point of speaking to the filmmaker and her mom and dad at the reception, but only because I had found the documentary so informative, honest, and poignant. I never dreamed it might be a portent of my future.

Chapter 4

Closed Captioning

E ntertainment options shrink when a person's hearing fails. The typical multiplex cranks up movie soundtracks to earth-shaking levels, but louder isn't necessarily better. If anything, what was left of my left-ear hearing was especially sensitive to high-decibel noise, and I didn't want to risk further damage. Athens has but one theater that occasionally screens a foreign film with subtitles, and while I do enjoy an occasional Swedish or French flick, I am partial to English-speaking movies. Which led me back to television, the medium on which I was raised and from which I made my living for many years after selling shoes and reading meters for the power company didn't work out.

The electronic media was my beat at the *Orlando Sentinel* in 1979, when the technology to create closed captions for TV programs was introduced and the nonprofit National Captioning Institute was launched. I went to a demonstration of the new, much-ballyhooed system and wrote a column about it for the paper. I explained how, if you had the proper device wired into your TV set, you could call up the sort of subtitles you'd see in a theater of a screening of a foreign film.

Neither my home nor office TV sets at the time had the new technology, however, and both my ears still worked just fine, so I never really got around to testing the system on an everyday basis.

I just assumed it worked exactly as publicized. Even years later, when I had a caption-capable set, the only time I ever turned it on was occasionally while watching *Masterpiece Theatre* on PBS. The sound quality on British imports such as *Upstairs, Downstairs* and *I, Claudius* was notoriously poor back then. Moreover, while the lords and ladies' stage diction rang clear enough, some of the servants' accents were so thick, they might as well have been speaking Scottish Gaelic. I made use of the captioning feature any time I encountered Dickens, Shakespeare, or Bob Hoskins, and I was ever so grateful.

Now that I found myself needing captioning all the time, I discovered an aggravating truth: some of the time it flat out sucks.

To be sure, closed captioning is a great boon to the deaf and hearing impaired, a godsend really. Yet there are times when I have found no captions preferable, times when the crawl on-screen should say, "Closed Captioned in Bulgarian." There are times when the on-screen end credit should say the captioning is provided by a grant from the Daffy Duck Foundation or the Marx Brothers Trust or, on particularly frustrating, diabolical occasions, the Joker. Times when the choice is between turn off the "CC" or throw a shoe at your flat-screen.

That's not really surprising when you're talking about live programming such as sporting events and news reports. The frequency of unusual names and technical terms is bound to result in errors, especially if the captions are being generated by voice-recognition software.

But the quality of captions for prerecorded programs also varied sharply. PBS, presumably because of its civic mission and its older-skewing audience, was the best and most consistent. Not only do its signature shows—*Masterpiece, Nature, NOVA*—boast exceptionally reliable captions, but it's rare to encounter mangled captions, let alone gibberish, on any of its dramas, documentaries, or investigative reports, as well.

Among commercial networks, CBS tended to be the most reliable, owing no doubt to awareness of an older core audience. *60 Minutes* is meticulously captioned, right down to the promos and correspondent intros. And popular CBS entertainment series such as *The Big Bang Theory*, *NCIS*, and *Blue Bloods* rarely have enough captioning glitches to be distracting.

At the other end of the spectrum were ABC and Fox, both of which court younger audiences. I'm not talking about misspelled words or translating "cruel" as "gruel." I'm talking about alphabetical train wrecks. The captioning of *Modern Family*, ABC's most acclaimed comedy and its most broadly appealing, was sometimes so incomprehensibly botched that it might have been medieval runes. Likewise, *The Simpsons*, Fox's immortal animated comedy, which is not only produced in South Korea, but also seemed at times to have been captioned in Korean, as well.

The DVD versions and syndicated reruns of these and other caption-impaired shows have accurate captions. If you don't mind waiting a few months to a year to see what your friends saw last night, you'll be able to understand every line.

Well, maybe. By the time I started writing this book, closed captioning had started to be more consistent and less error-prone, but a new problem for the hearing impaired had emerged: speed.

TV storytelling had always tended to be more talky and less visual than movies, but the splintering of the viewing audience by cable and streaming services has left platforms and producers obsessively time-conscious, fearful of short attention spans. Thus, the talk on TV is increasingly turbocharged.

Sitcoms that had once been paced like stage plays took on the frantic feel of 1930s screwball comedies like *His Gal Friday* and *Bringing Up Baby*. If *All in the Family* was Archie Bunker's old LaSalle doing forty-five mph, *Modern Family* is a BMW zipping along at seventy. The back-and-forth on cable-news cage matches like *Tucker Carlson Tonight* and *The Rachel Maddow Show* is as dizzying as Olympic ping-pong. Even the broadcast networks' early-evening newscasts, though the commercials for drugs and denture adhesives indicate an awareness of an older audience, have taken on a breathless pace (yes, I'm talking about you, David "Breaking News!" Muir). Only a speed-reader can keep up, and even then, it's often at the expense of the images flashing by. You "watch" TV or you read it. It's hard to do both.

The best alternatives I've found are old Western movies with long takes on mountain vistas and slower-talking stars like John Wayne and Jimmy Stewart. I've even tried pretalkies, reacquainting myself with the genius of Harold Lloyd and Buster Keaton. And then there are books. Hearing loss will make a person renew his or her library card.

Chapter 5

Wicked

By the middle of June, three months after my ear wreck, it was clear that methotrexate was having little discernible impact on my hearing loss. I might experience a slight, encouraging gain midday only to have it disappear by dinnertime, or I would experience no gain at all. I was sleeping poorly, a side effect of the drug I'd been warned about. One night, when I was sleeping soundly, I was startled out of slumber by what sounded like the shrieking sound effect that accompanies the notorious shower scene in *Psycho*. It wasn't the alarm on my bedroom clock radio going off or a car alarm on the street in front of our house. It was just my sound-starved ears having a little fun.

I was weary and low-energy, unsure whether I was reacting to medication or truly depressed. The new normal for me hearing-wise was good enough to detect rattling cutlery in the silverware drawer or the coffee grinder's grating whine, little more. The cruder the sound, it seemed, the easier. An audiologist told me this was because crude sound, unlike conversational speech or music, requires only that we recognize it. We don't have to extract any meaning from it.

Other than having people write me notes on a steno pad, text messaging was by default my main means of communication. Downie Winkler, my stepdaughter, had shamed me into belatedly adopting the thumb-typing cell-phone system so essential to her generation and so often much ridiculed by me. Now texting was my lifeline. Not only did Marty and I text back and forth while I was at the Peabody office, but we also occasionally texted inside our house. It was easier sometimes for her than flipping lights on and off to get my attention or throwing a ball of rolled-up socks at me.

At the office, I had Marty record a message on UGA's automated answering system advising potential entrants, network publicists, and salespeople that "Noel Holston, public relations coordinator of the Peabody Awards, is currently dealing with a hearing loss and would much appreciate it if you would contact him at his email address."

My colleagues, even those whose offices adjoined mine, largely stopped sticking their heads in my door or trying to chat. They just emailed.

I couldn't participate in phone conversations or hear messages left on my machine. I couldn't make a haircut appointment by phone, order pizza, or tell a telemarketer to get lost. Radio was a no-go. TV worked for me only with crap-shoot closed captioning. Face-to-face conversation was almost impossible with anyone but Marty, and even she was beginning to lose patience.

I was already notorious in my family for my tendency to space out and miss social cues. Now, mired in my growing frustration, I did not appreciate how taxing it was to be around me for more than a few minutes at a time. Conversation is like breathing to Marty. When she's with a group of friends or her brothers and sisters—she's one of fourteen siblings—the talk is like a jazz jam, with swoops and sudden segues. Our first meeting had been an invigorating jab-ber-fest. Our marriage was an ongoing conversation, a free-form discussion of life, spirituality, politics, and art, a rat-a-tat exchange of banter, barbs, asides, and puns. Now we were on the level of "See Spot run."

She bought me an American Sign Language picture book and started teaching me the sign alphabet. She had learned the ABCs and some basic ASL phrases when she read *The Miracle Worker* in a high-school English class. I practiced, protesting all the while that I knew no one particularly well, excepting her, who was even moderately conversant in ASL, and that if I were no better at learning sign than I'd been at Spanish or French, it would be years before we could have anything resembling a lively conversation. She finger-spelled an expression I will not quote in a family-friendly book. I got busy working on my ABCs.

* * *

Dr. Fishman told me, through Marty, to discontinue the methotrexate. He sent us back to Dr. Steenerson, who said he was stymied and out of options, save one: a cochlear implant.

I was open to the idea of getting a bionic ear; I'd read about it in science magazines and done a bit of internet research. Marty was game, as well. There was one slight hitch. Dr. Steenerson was not in the pool of physicians covered by my Blue Cross Blue Shield HMO plan. Out-of-network office visits were one thing. We could bite the bullet and pay $250-$300 out of pocket for the services of a specialist like him. But a cochlear implant operation could set us back. Way back. For the same amount of money an implant operation would cost, we could buy a new BMW and a Ford Expedition SUV and still have enough change left for a week's vacation in Paris and a jumbo bag of M&Ms. Even in the best of times, that would have been a gargantuan bullet to bite. But this was June 2010, two years after the burst housing bubble and the ensuing stock market dive had ravaged our retirement savings.

We told Dr. Steenerson that as much as we would prefer to have him operate—he was, after all, a cochlear-surgery pioneer and widely considered the best in the Southeast at his specialty—we'd have to find someone in our insurance network to perform the implantation. He said he understood and had one of his office staff provide us with a list of other cochlear surgeons in the Atlanta area.

We settled on Dr. Karen Hoffmann of Piedmont ENT, a large, thriving practice in an upscale section of Atlanta called Buckhead. She was relatively young but had performed hundreds of implantations. Reviews of her work online were glowing. And she was covered by my Blue Cross plan. We liked her, and the clinic's nurses and office staff were sympathetic and friendly.

Dr. Hoffmann surprised us, however, by not scheduling me for surgery immediately. She said she had another treatment she'd like to try first, something new, a sort of hearing Hail Mary pass. Theorizing that the oral steroid that I had taken had diminishing impact because it was too diffused, she wanted to put a "micro wick," a tiny stent, in the eardrum of my right ear. Through it, I would apply Dexamethasone ear drops directly to my middle ear, three times a day.

"If it doesn't work," she said, "we'll schedule the implant surgery for fall."

I said sure, what the heck. I already have a pierced ear. Might as well have a pierced eardrum. I'll be a guinea pig. I would just as well not have her—or any other doctor—bore a hole in my skull and wire up my cochlea.

Thus began a month of dribbling the liquid corticosteroid into my ear morning, noon, and night and lying on my side for ten to fifteen minutes while it dripped into my middle ear and, seemingly, into my brain itself. I was instructed not to swim, period, and to stay out of the shower until I got a custom ear plug to seal the ear canal off. I also had to chase the Dexamethasone drops with antibacterial Ofloxacin drops to minimize the chance of infection around the wick. It made me think of the old folk song about an old woman who swallowed a fly, then a succession of larger critters, and lastly a horse. She died, of course, but I tried not to dwell on that.

During this experiment, my tinnitus, a problem off and on for years, reached new highs. And lows. And attained sound effects that I could never have imagined.

Nature is said to abhor a vacuum. The human ear and brain abhor silence. If auditory stimulation from the outside world is cut off, the brain and the ear will make up for it, creating phantom sounds usually labeled tinnitus. Though it's sometimes used interchangeably with "ringing in the ears," tinnitus can in fact take many forms, from beeping and squeaking to buzzing and shrieking. It can also be impressively complex. Midsummer, my tinnitus went into overdrive. Perhaps because I had spent so much of my life immersed in music—dancing to it, cooking to it, driving to it, making love to it—my tinnitus often had a symphonic element.

Years of reporting and columnizing on a daily basis had made writing reflexive for me. I try not to let any experience go to waste. To paraphrase an old saying, that which doesn't kill you makes for a good story. So, in August, I composed an essay about my crazy tinnitus. It was published on www.likethedew.com, a Georgia-based website. The Dew is officially "A journal of progressive Southern culture & politics," but founder Lee Leslie grants regular contributors like myself some leeway so long as we're Dixie bred.

This is what I posted under the headline "Radio Head":

Since my ears stopped working almost six months ago, I've heard a ton of music. But I don't mean that I've been summoning up old favorite recordings from memory, although I am fortunate enough to be able to do that. I can "play" most of the Beatles' canon and dozens of albums in my head anytime I care to, more or less whole.

I'm talking about music that my brain and my sickly inner ears generate entirely on their own. Spontaneously. Electro-chemically. Unstoppably.

For the past couple of weeks, pretty much every minute I was awake, I heard a tune strongly reminiscent of "Telstar," the instrumental by the Tornados that became a chart-topper in 1962 thanks to its "weird" space-age sound.

Now, you may be thinking, "Good grief, 'Telstar' 24/7—it's a wonder he hasn't drowned himself yet." But the thing is, I'm a glass half-full kind of a guy. If I have to have a moldy-oldie instrumental looping through my head, I would prefer something that sounds more like the Chantays' "Pipeline" or Duke Ellington's "East St. Louis Toodle-oo." But I am very grateful I'm not stuck with, oh, the Champs' "Tequila" or Paul Muriat's "Love Is Blue." Well, not yet anyway.

The riffs running through my head have a tendency to change unpredictably. For a while, it was an unfamiliar progression of bass notes. For another while, it was something that sounded kind of like Nancy Wilson's roaring, power-chord intro to Heart's "Crazy on You." And yet another while, in a rare classical interlude, it was like "March of the Wooden Soldiers" from The Nutcracker. More than once I caught myself in mid-strut with a garden rake or a broom over my shoulder as the family cat, Cadbury, observed me with more than his usual disdain.

According to my research, I have been experiencing "musical hallucinations," a variation of tinnitus, the phantom sounds often heard by people whose hearing is going, going or gone. The Mayo Clinic website lists half a dozen common tinnitus "sounds": ringing, buzzing, roaring, clicking, whistling, hissing.

Each of these is an old friend now, but the single-word designations don't do my experience justice. There are times when I wonder if I have a phantom Phil Spector in my head, overproducing my tinnitus variations in his famous "Wall of Sound" style.

At various times, I hear:

Torrents of Spring—Raging, rushing water, occasionally punctuated by what sounds like a frightened animal being swept away.

Red River—Not to be confused with *Torrents of Spring*, this is the sound of a stampede, like the thundering, climactic cow-panic in the classic John Wayne Western.

747—Not like you hear inside the big jet; like what the ground crew would hear if they took off their ear mufflers.

Hearts of Space—Reminiscent of what you'd hear on the long-running, late-night radio series devoted to New Age, ambient and electronic "space" music, it's sweeping, free-form sound, like something from an old Isao Tomita album, interrupted by gurgles, beeps and the arcing sonic equivalent of shooting stars.

Factory Floor—An industrial cacophony.

These variations of tinnitus do not necessarily take turns manifesting themselves. I may "hear," for instance, *Torrents of Spring* in one ear and *Factory Floor* in the other while that "Telstar"-like riff or the "Wooden Soldiers" theme is also audible. And while this is all going on, entirely beyond my control, I can consciously recall an entirely different song or a harmony.

Once again, you may be wondering how it is that I haven't drowned myself yet. Well, as I said, I'm a glass half-full kind of guy. I'm hopeful. If, according to the laws of probability, a monkey might hunt-and-peck *Hamlet* given enough time and typing paper, then one of these days all the sounds in my head might come together and I will have composed something akin to Tchaikovsky's "1812 Overture."

*   *   *

I include the piece here in the hope that it illustrates a crucial point that I was learning about coping with the various and sundry manifestations and ramifications of severe hearing loss: if you can't maintain a sense of humor, you are in deep trouble.

Chapter 6

I'd Rather Go Blind

Being seriously hearing impaired means you have to be on guard constantly not to allow yourself to become isolated, choosing a solitary existence simply because socializing is so much work. It's okay to grieve your loss, but you can't allow grieving to sour and settle into depression and retreat.

Still, with my social circle steadily shrinking and the sounds in my head going cuckoo, I was moving up the Kubler-Ross scale to anger, the whole "Why me?" thing. I felt as though I had trod pretty lightly on this Earth, not causing a lot of harm that I was aware of. I drive an economy car. I compost. I recycle. I send checks regularly to PBS, the Salvation Army, and the American Society for the Prevention of Cruelty to Animals. So why was I losing my auditory function while Osama bin Laden could still hear the call to daily prayers? And why, of all senses, my hearing, when music and lively conversation were like air to me?

I wanted to make a swap-and-trade of my deafness for blindness. If I never saw another sunset, I told myself, I would deal with it. Better that than never again hearing music that moved my feet and touched my soul. Tom Petty once told an interviewer that music was "probably the only real magic" he had ever experienced in life.

"It's pure and it's real," he said. "And it moves and it heals and it communicates and does all these incredible things."[1]

Its power had buoyed me, doctored me, transported me, and saved me more times than I could count.

What if I never again heard Louis Armstrong raise glorious ruckuses with his Hot Fives or Lucinda Williams describe a suicide's sad funeral in "Pineola"? What if I never again heard my wife?

I met Marty in March of 1993, when I was starting to dabble in songwriting and decided I needed a collaborator. I thought my lyrics were pretty clever, but my tunes were about as imaginative as "Row, Row, Row Your Boat." I made a list of musicians, male and female, whom I had encountered professionally as a journalist in Minneapolis covering arts and entertainment. One after another, I treated them to lunch or brunch, talked tunesmithery with them, and showed them some of my lyrics. Marty was the sixth or seventh musician I dined with. She was the founder of an all-female a cappella group, The Collective, and she'd sent me a shmooze note after I mentioned the band laudably in a *Star Tribune* feature story I had done the year before about the local cabaret scene.

I had filed her note away. I wasn't sure which one of the group members she was. Turned out, she was the little one with the short, short hair. When I arrived at The Egg and I, a popular south Minneapolis breakfast joint, I scanned the room and spotted a woman I was pretty sure was she. Her outfit that frigid Minnesota morning was a silver-gray, one-piece snow suit that made her look as rotund as the Michelin Man. When she saw me standing by the door, she recognized me from my *Star Tribune* mugshot. She flashed a sunburst smile that could melt a glacier. We ate the "kamikaze pancakes"—lumberjack-worthy buckwheat slabs bulked up with fruit and nuts—and yakked about music and life. She was juggling being

---

1   Neil McCormick, "Tom Petty: A rock star for the ages," *The Telegraph,* June 16, 2012, https://www.telegraph.co.uk/culture/music /rockandpopfeatures/9334051/Tom-Petty-a-rock-star-for-the-ages.html.

a single mom with her band gigs and a day job as house mother at a group home for mentally handicapped/mentally ill adults. I gave her a short stack of my lyrics when we headed for our respective cars.

"You talk . . . good," I stammered as we said good-bye.

"I talk 'good'?" she laughed. "You call yourself a professional writer?" she jibed in response to my grammatical error.

I was intrigued. I was also married. Not happily, but married nonetheless. Three years earlier, my wife had told me she wanted out of our marriage of seventeen years. She said she was deeply unhappy and needed to find herself. We had married right after I finished college. She had dropped out of school and was working at Disney World. All our friends were getting hitched. Why not us? It seemed like the normal, proper thing to do. We were young and dumb. We didn't know our own selves, much less each other. The biggest surprise about our breakup was that it didn't come sooner.

Clair and I had the big sit-down with our sons, Damon, sixteen, and Alexander, thirteen, and told them what was coming. Clair planned to get an apartment, finish getting her second college degree, in chemistry, and make a new life. I would take over primary parenting. We found a buyer for the big, money-pit house we'd naively picked out when we moved to Minneapolis in 1986. We purchased a smaller, cheaper house in the same school district so as not to disrupt the boys' lives any more than we already were.

As moving day drew near, Clair got cold feet about striking out on her own. She asked if she could move into the new house with me and the boys. Our estrangement didn't end, however, and the tension between us grew steadily unbearable. I wrote a song about how I was meeting women who interested me, women I would notice but not try for. The opening lyrics:

I'm my own worst enemy
I'm gonna be the death of me
I'm falling in love and I'm not free
I've gotta stop breakin' my own heart

That's the state I was in when I brunched with Marty that morning.

We began creating music together. We discovered our voices blended nicely (although, in truth, with her three-and-a-half octave range and her flawless ear for harmony, she could make Tom Waits or Mr. Ed sound mellifluous). Our first gig—I had never in my life played a "gig"—was an AIDS-research fundraiser in Minneapolis's Minnehaha Park. We worked up a short set with some of her musician buddies: the Beatles' "I've Just Seen A Face," the Everly Brothers' "Bye Bye Love," a couple of my songs, and one of hers. Clair and our son Xan attended. Marty and I were still in denial.

One morning soon thereafter, I drove by her house on the way to work and pushed a note and a lyric sheet under her front door. The lyrics were to the aforementioned "I've Gotta Stop Breakin' My Own Heart." I'd finally polished up the verses but still had only a clunky melody. A day later, when I got to work at the *Star Tribune* and checked my messages, I heard Marty's voice, singing the song. The beautiful, wistful melody she'd heard in my words made me gasp.

Three months later, I moved out of my house. Too uncertain (and broke) to rent an apartment, I became a serial house sitter, moving from colleague's apartment to vacationing friend's home. Eventually, Clair told me our original split-up plan was the right idea: she would find an apartment, and I would move back into our house and take care of the boys. Meanwhile, Marty and I were becoming an item, romantically as well as musically.

I had sung for as long as I could remember—in church choirs, at parties, in a folk group in Minneapolis, and in community theater productions of *The Music Man, Working*, and other musicals. But this was different. A new world opened up to me, and music became an essential element of my partnership with Marty. I joined her onstage to sing songs of hers, mine, and ours at bars, coffee houses, and clubs all over the Twin Cities—Ball's, The Fine Line, The Dakota—and later, when I went to work for *Newsday*, at venues on Long Island. I sang backup on her albums, and one of our songs became a favorite of Great American Songbook expert Jonathan Schwartz, who played Marty regularly on his WNYC radio broadcasts in New York. One Saturday, as I was driving on the LI Expressway, he played an album cut of hers on which she and I traded verses. I was so joyously thunderstruck hearing myself singing on the radio that I almost had a wreck.

After we moved to Georgia, Marty eventually succeeded in getting me to take my abilities more seriously. I started recording a CD of my own using her producer. I had three finished tracks in the can when my hearing collapsed. Singing ceased to be an option. I could still kind of carry a tune if I knew it well and sang all by my lonesome, but pair me with any instrument or another singer, and what came out of my mouth was fit only for empty halls, shower stalls, and dog pounds. Marty and I had often sung "Happy Birthday" duets on the phone to faraway relatives and friends. Now, when I would attempt to join her, she would give me a sad, sympathetic smile and mouth, "No."

I wanted sound, musical sound, back in my life. A chorus, a chorus, my kingdom for a chorus!

How I missed harmony. Much as I enjoyed singing by myself—singing in the shower, singing along with records—there was nothing like joining voices with another person or persons. With Marty and with the old-time music ensemble that I was part of in Minneapolis, I was blessed to occasionally produce blends, chords, that were at once physical and metaphysical, that unleashed swells of positive feelings in my chest, that had a euphoric effect, buoyant, therapeutic, invigorating, holy. Would I ever be so lucky again?

In the chapter about hearing in her book *A Natural History of the Senses,* Diane Ackerman wrote that "Sounds thicken the sensory stew of our lives, and we depend on them to help us interpret, communicate with and express the world around us."[2]

In *Rebuilt: How Becoming Part Computer Made Me More Human*, cochlear implantee Michael Chorost contends that hearing "constitutes your sense of being *of* the world, in the thick of it. To see is to observe, but to hear is to be enveloped."[3]

While reading up on famous people who've suffered hearing loss—Ludwig von Beethoven, Pete Townsend, Huey Lewis, Rush Limbaugh—I ran across a quote from Helen Keller, the subject of the play and movie *The Miracle Worker* and the poster woman for triumphing over adversity. She contended that deafness was "a much worse misfortune" than blindness because "it means the loss of the most vital stimulus—the sound of the voice that brings language, sets thoughts astir and keeps us in the intellectual company of man."

I mentioned this to Marty. Her initial response was to remind me that Ms. Keller "didn't have the benefit of emails or texting or chat rooms."

Then she set me straight with uncharacteristic harshness.

"Don't you let me ever hear you say that again," she said.

She reminded me that she had been a volunteer reader for the blind back at the time we first met. "You have no idea how completely blindness would transform your life, how much it would limit you," she said. "Deafness is a frustration. It's an inconvenience. But you can still drive a car. You can still shop at the grocery store. You have no clue how difficult your life would be. Don't *ever* say that."

I got her point. And after I thought it through, I *really* got her point.

---

2   Diane Ackerman, *A Natural History of the Senses* (New York: Random House, 1990), 175.
3   Michael Chorost, *Rebuilt: How Becoming Part Computer Made Me More Human* (New York: Houghton Mifflin Company, 2005), 9.

Besides, there are no trades to be had. You deal with the disability you're dealt or you don't.

You have to find the absurdity in your situation, laugh about the hated, crazy-making song that's playing on your cochlear stereo, and snicker over the misheard phrases. Did you say we should go to "golf shoes"? No, it was Gulf Shores. Do I want to "grind the faraway beads"? No, rye with caraway seeds.

And you have to not only learn the basics of minimizing your disadvantage, but you also have to put them into practice.

Chapter 7
Sitting Here in Limbo

The longer I struggled with hearing that veered from poor to almost nonexistent, the more I appreciated that deafness is a disability of degree. People who are fully without hearing function, and people who were born deaf or have suffered some sort of catastrophic loss early in life, have a community. Indeed, they *are* a community. They're the Deaf with a capital D, a societal subset united by their common disability and the coping mechanisms, notably sign language, that they have developed over decades to address and minimize it.

Some profoundly deaf people interact regularly with the hearing world. Perhaps the most famous modern example is Marlee Matlin. Not only hasn't she allowed deafness to deter her from pursuing an acting career, but she has put her lip-reading ability, fluency in sign language, and arduously acquired speaking ability to effective use in film roles that include *Children of a Lesser God*, for which she won an Academy Award. Other profoundly deaf people, for various reasons, gravitate to other deaf people.

At the *Star Tribune* in Minneapolis, where I was a columnist and feature writer from 1986 to 2001, there was a group of typesetters who were profoundly deaf. Encouraging hiring of the deaf was a printer's union tradition at newspapers in larger cities. The deaf workers maintained their own tables in a back corner of the *Star*

Tribune's cafeteria. I would often notice a group of them signing animatedly and laughing loudly and wonder what the joke was.

The significant but not complete hearing loss that I was experiencing—and that is the most common—is not like that. It offers no community. You're neither here nor there. You're in no-man's-land, limbo.

It's often like being at a dinner gathering in a foreign country with whose native tongue you are just minimally familiar—only a smattering of words and phrases. You listen with all the concentration you can muster, hoping to catch a complete word you recognize, all the while looking for clues in the speaker's inflection and body language. You shift your gaze from side to side as if you were watching a tennis match, hoping everyone won't talk at once and create a conversational sonic boom, hoping the table won't erupt in laughter.

It encourages withdrawal, isolation, and that's a gravitational pull I knew I must resist. It's exhausting, with most every social occasion a marathon, a gauntlet. But it has to be run. The only option is drop out, retire. If I hadn't had a wife who has refused to let me go AWOL, I might well have become an auditory hermit.

One of the insights hearing impairment has given me is how uncomfortable most American men are with physical closeness. I realize now that I was one of them before my hearing loss. I hugged women friends hello and good-bye but shook men friends' hands—or embraced them so lightly we barely felt the contact and slapped them on the back robustly to prove I was just a hale and hearty fellow. I snickered at Frenchmen and Italians in movies kissing each other's cheeks and rolled my eyes when World Cup soccer players piled upon one another in orgies of congratulation after a goal.

Once I understood the importance of getting up close and personal with whoever was speaking to me (the better to minimize words evaporating into the ether), and looking them squarely in the mouth (the better to read their lips), I began to put these revelations into practice. I noticed that many people became uneasy and pulled back if I got closer than two feet from them. The two male colleagues at work that I most needed to interact with invariably took a step back if I leaned in in hopes of understanding their words better. It quickly became routine for us to converse by email, even though we had adjoining offices.

Friends, even well-meaning, sympathetic ones, drifted away. One of the best guy pals I had made since moving to Athens, a fellow with whom I shared passions for politics, the NBA, and music, initially made a concerted effort to proceed as if nothing had happened. We would get together for coffee or lunch, and he would write out his side of our conversation on a legal pad or text me his answers even though we were three feet apart. As the months wore on, however, our coffee dates got farther and farther apart. Then there were none. I understood. I had become a lot of work, slower on the uptake, and less fun. I couldn't really blame him.

My own sons, especially the older, Damon, already impatient by nature, struggled with the tediousness of communicating with me. At times it must have felt to him as if he were out on the highway and stuck behind an old coot who was driving thirty miles per hour in a fifty-five zone. My younger son, Alexander, handled it somewhat better. I asked Xan why he was more patient. He wrote tellingly on a pad, "Because I'm the father of a three-year old."

In the other extreme, there were people like my friend Kathleen Ryan. A massage therapist, she's accustomed to close physical contact. Touch is second nature to her, so much so that she occasionally startles new acquaintances with spontaneous shoulder rubs. She also has hearing issues herself, wearing aids in both ears. She understands that when

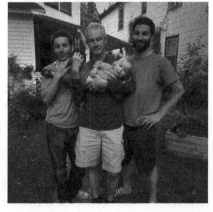

Photo courtesy of Alice Kirchhoff

she's conversing with me, she needs to speak up, not LOUDLY but clearly, and to use good diction and not put her hand in front of her mouth.

More Kathleens in my life would have been a great boon, but they weren't easy to find. Deafness is not only a disability of degree, but it's also largely an invisible disability. The deaf and hearing impaired don't bob their heads like Stevie Wonder or wear impenetrably dark sunglasses or tap-test their paths with white canes. Other than looking lost at times or glancing around feverishly trying to compensate for the absence of sound cues with vision, they—we, I should say—look pretty normal. It's estimated that nearly forty million Americans, kids and teens as well as seniors, have some level of hearing loss. I personally know only a handful of them.

It's a disability that can be hidden, at least in the short term, and most hearing-impaired people don't hesitate to try. To acknowledge deafness can be risky. You may be perceived as older, slower, or dumber. Katherine Bouton, author of *Shouting Won't Help: Why I—and 50 Million Other Americans—Can't Hear You*, actually gave up her job as an editor at the *New York Times* because she couldn't bring herself to explain to management that she had not become incompetent or antisocial, just seriously hearing impaired.[4]

My stepdaughter Downie confided to her mother that I seemed to have lost a dozen IQ points. It's painful to be told that, but I got it. Sitting at my computer, I felt I'd never been sharper mentally. Sitting on the living room sofa, I couldn't chew gum and listen at the same time. I expended so much energy and focus just trying to sort out what people were saying, comments and comebacks occurred to me long after the subject had changed.

Sometimes I would raise my hand or clear my throat, interrupt the conversational flow, and say something like, "Can we backtrack

---

4   Katherine Bouton, *Shouting Won't Help: Why I—and 50 Million Other Americans,—Can't Hear You* (New York: Sarah Crichton Books, FSG, 2013), 186–187.

for just a moment?" I would reintroduce a topic, add the thought or the information that had come to me belatedly, and then tighten my jaw, flex my ears, and prepare to try to capture the response as if I were getting ready to deadlift a hefty barbell. Sometimes it helped. Other times, I was just reminded that, hearing-wise, I was now the proverbial ninety-eight-pound weakling.

Chapter 8

Pride and Prejudice

I almost titled this book *Deaf Be Not Proud*, and not just because I have seldom met a pun I didn't like. If you are dealing with a substantial hearing loss, you can't afford to be proud or vain. Rule number one for coping is:

Do Not Try to Hide Your Disability

It will only make things worse.

There will be people who will judge you if you have a visible hearing aid or cochlear implant. They may presume you are older than you are. Or slower. Or dumber. Or less capable. You could say, "Well, that's their problem," and that's true. But it's also yours, and you have to deal with it.

You need to take a pad and pen with you wherever you go—and not be embarrassed to use it.

You need to do your eating out earlier, if possible, before restaurants get more crowded and noisy.

You need to ask for tables on the edges of dining rooms, a corner if possible, and give yourself the seat that puts your back against a wall, minimizing the surrounding buzz.

And you have to become a coach of sorts. You have to explain the new ground rules. Most people, even family and friends, don't know what to do instinctively besides talk louder. Loudness is in fact more likely to reduce a hearing-impaired person's comprehension of speech.

Rude as it may seem, you have to ask people to make sure they have your full attention before they start talking. If you are seriously hearing impaired, there's no such thing as casual conversation. You can't hear out of "the corner of your ear." You probably can't listen while doing any chore that requires focus. Missing just two or three words at the beginning of someone's comment to you can leave you to play a hopeless game of catch-up. Context is paramount.

You have to ask people to look directly at you when they are speaking to you. Even if you can't speechread (the new term for lipreading), there are clues in a speaker's expressions and body language that you don't even have to be actively aware of to incorporate into your understanding. We hear with our eyes, too.

If you are part of a group gathering, you have to ask people to speak one at a time.

This last is not easy. Even friends with the best of intentions often get carried away in the excitement of a conversation and forget your request. It's not natural to take turns.

In the first months of my hearing loss, when various drugs were producing wild swings, nothing made me want to pull my hair out, bang my head on the table, or just walk away, alone, more than Happy Hour.

Athens, often cited as one of the great college towns in America, is a place where drinking is an activity almost as popular as breathing. Soon after Marty and I moved to Athens, a couple of old friends invited us to be part of their Happy Hour group, a floating gaggle of fifteen to twenty people—university faculty and staff, musicians, an ER doctor, a carpenter, a city attorney—who got together at one of the town's many bars around six on Friday nights to have a Terrapin (the local microbrew) or a Pabst Blue Ribbon and shoot the breeze about their workweek, politics, music, and the world. The conversations were fast, funny, and profane. Topics could change in a heartbeat. I loved these gatherings. Many times we walked away from Max Canada or The Go Bar toward a nearby soul food or pizza emporium saying, "God, I love this town."

I still loved Athens after my hearing loss, but Happy Hour? Not so much. Even at an outdoor patio table with less surrounding noise, trying to keep up with a conversation that jumped like an eight-way air hockey match was challenging and ultimately defeating. You listen so hard it strains your brain. Your eyes dart this way and that, constantly, looking for lip movement to go with what sound you do hear. Occasionally, you catch a phrase you recognize, but by the time you extrapolate a larger thought or sentence from it and think up a comment or retort, the conversation has shifted or moved on. If you're feeling assertive, you will raise your hand, like you're a kid in class, and ask if could take the conversation back a few seconds, rewind, and offer your thought on the topics. Sometimes it will add to the conversation. Sometimes you'll realize you misheard what was said and that your comment is a non sequitur. Sometimes you will just sip your beer and laugh anytime you see other people at the table laughing.

You have to brief people about how to talk to you if they expect you to grasp what they're saying. And you have to be pushy enough to remind them when they almost invariably forget. Even my brother, after dealing professionally with the deaf and hard of hearing for four decades, forgets. Whenever I visit him in Mobile, at some point I will have to remind him that he can't run water in the kitchen sink while he's talking to me or turn on an electric can opener. A healthy ear is a multitasking marvel, capable of selectively sifting an amazing array of sonic input. Mine, alas, had become a masked marvel.

Chapter 9

Location, Location, Location

The microwick Dr. Hoffmann had placed in my right eardrum was no more successful than the methotrexate. After two months of my dutifully drizzling steroid drops directly down my ear canal without any lasting impact, Dr. Hoffmann told me to discontinue the treatment and start thinking seriously about a cochlear implant. The more immediate issue for me, however, was my younger son's wedding in Minneapolis, set for early August. I asked Dr. Hoffmann if she could give me a fresh prescription of the oral Prednisone that, with luck, would give me a temporary hearing boost that would enable me to hear the vows and make conversation.

I started taking the drug the day before Marty and I flew north, trying to time it so that the peak of my steroid-fueled hearing would coincide with the big day. The strategy was moderately successful. Conversations over drinks or dinner were the usual frustrating trial, but I made myself relish opportunities just to be in the spirit of the banter among Alexander and his partner-to-be, Morgen, and my older son, Damon, and his wife, Alice, and their friends. Even if the chatter was too quick and random for me to follow, it was sweet just to watch their expressions and soak up their high spirits. And when we were in a car, zipping around Minneapolis picking up their suits at the tailor's and shopping for cool socks and suspenders, I could understand a good bit of what was said.

The wedding itself was like a pantomime play. An outdoor affair, set up at the foot of an historic stone bridge across the Mississippi River, it was unintelligible. When Xan and Morgen exchanged vows, the words evaporated into the open air. I had to be content to watch their lips move and see their smiles.

At the reception afterward, I was asked to make a toast. Thanks as much to the miracle of bone conduction of sound in my skull as to the Prednisone, I could hear what I said. Later on, the newlyweds sent me a copy of the vows I couldn't hear.

I also got to see, if not quite hear, Marty perform that week at the Minneapolis Fringe Festival, a showcase for dance, music, and other performing arts, often as not quirky and irreverent. Backed by guitarist Tate Ferguson and Kate Bordeaux, one of her Collective bandmates, she sang live accompaniment for new works by two different dance companies. For one, she performed "At Last," "Sunday Kind of Love," and other Etta James songs. The other company created dances to songs of hers—and ours.

The worst moment of the trip was when I yelled at her while she was driving. She had missed a turn and I went ballistic. She forgave me, but she said it was only because she knew I was on steroids.

I determined that after I got home, I was done with steroids for good. I would leave 'roid rage to the professional athletes.

The trip home was like a movie, too. An absurdist comedy. A *Monty Python* sketch.

Marty stayed on in Minneapolis for another music gig. I flew back accompanied by my stepdaughter. What made airport security in Minneapolis search me, I still can't figure. Maybe they were picking passengers at random. Maybe they thought I was a particularly wily terrorist who had mastered the art of disguising himself as a sleep-deprived, middle-aged bozo in cargo shorts who had partied too hard at his son's wedding reception. Maybe they thought the big red "C" on my *Colbert Report* baseball cap stood for Communist. Maybe it's because hearing impairment can make you seem odd and thus suspicious.

They were after me from the moment I showed my Georgia driver's license and got my boarding pass scribbled on. A TSA agent spoke to me and motioned with his hands palm up.

I said, "I'm sorry, sir, I can't hear." He reemphasized the gesture emphatically, the hand-signal equivalent of yelling. I said, "I'm sorry, I don't know what you want me to do."

I suggested he talk to my traveling companion, Downie, who is biracial and doesn't look remotely like me. "She can translate," I said.

He ignored that and made the gesture again. I gestured back with what I would call my "I'm clueless" shrug. He grabbed me by both wrists and turned my palms up. Then he wiped each with some sort of napkin pad and motioned for me to move on.

I was thinking, "Well, that's the famous 'Minnesota nice' for ya. Them Norskies are makin' sure I don't catch a flu bug or something."

I proceeded to the conveyor belt, dumped my tennis shoes and change into a bin, and put my carry-on bag behind it. The guard at the walk-through scanner looked annoyed when I told him I couldn't understand his words, but he let me through. Then, as I went to collect my stuff, a grim-faced guard, a woman, said something to me.

Downie stepped in quickly this time: "He's deaf, ma'am." And then, to me, she mouthed, slowly: "She asked if she can search your bag."

I shrugged. Sure. Fine. No problem.

The woman put on protective latex gloves and used another of those wipes to rub around the inside of the bag. Then she tested what's on the wipe in a computerized machine that gave a readout. Downie and I were standing there rolling our eyes at each other, and other travelers were looking at us funny.

I was wondering, "Do they think I'm smuggling drugs?" I was wondering what on Earth caught their attention, and I was about to say, "If there's white powder, it's Gold Bond," when it hit me. I had a small can of shoe polish in the bag that I had neglected to transfer to my baggie of liquids.

The woman soon pulled out the little can, which was unfortunately wrapped up in the cloth I use to apply it. The shoe polish color was oxblood, so when she pulled the cloth out, it looked as though it might contain a severed finger or a bloody eyeball.

She gingerly carried it over to the X-ray, holding it at arm's length. She ran it through the machine, and after much deliberation, she and two other guards determined that, yes, it was a can of shoe polish. And I was thinking, "You know, you could have just asked."

Next, they ran my carry-on through X-ray again, presumably to be safe, and they got agitated all over again. She put my bag back on the table and rummaged through it, pulling out my blue boxer shorts embossed with images of penguins, a couple of Marty's CDs, my toothbrush, and the arch supports from my wedding shoes.

Finally, she carefully lifted an object out of the suitcase that, from a distance, looked as though it had wires sticking out of it. And I went, "Aha!"

It was a bolo tie, black and silver with a blue stone inset, that my father-in-law, Don Winkler, an auto mechanic-turned-jewelry maker in retirement, made for me.

What it obviously was, however, the guard didn't seem to grasp. Or maybe she was just following protocol. She unwrapped the tissue I had put around the stone to protect it and then, very carefully, as though it were a snake that might bite her, she took the bolo to the X-ray. After much deliberation, she and another TSA agent confirmed that it was indeed jewelry. She put it back in the bag and set the bag on a table. It now looked like raccoons had gone through it looking for grubs. She motioned to me. I indicated, again, that I am nearly deaf. She leaned over and said loudly in my left ear, "You're done!"

No "Thank you for your patience," no "Sorry," no sign of embarrassment. She just walked away.

I packed up, and Downie and I headed for our gate. Since we got no explanation, I can only guess how it might have looked to them: that the can of something semisolid and the bolo strings with metal tips were the makings of an explosive device.

Flying back to Atlanta, where the same "bomb fixings" had sailed through security without a word a few days earlier, I contemplated what a strange and inconsistent activity keeping us safe from underwear and shoe bombers is. And I realized I had been taught two valuable lessons about modern air travel:

- Deafness can foster behavior that makes you look furtive and shifty. Try not to dart your eyes around too much at airports.

- If you plan to accessorize with a dangerous bolo tie in another city, don't pack it, wear it.

*   *   *

Soon after Marty got back from Minneapolis, we drove to Atlanta yet again, this time to meet with Dr. Hoffmann and start making plans for the surgery. She surprised us by asking which of my ears I would prefer to have implanted. I had thought it obvious: the right ear, the one that we'd been trying to salvage. But she said the left, in which I still had a little natural hearing remaining, might be a better candidate.

I nixed that based on the marvelous, inexplicable fact that perhaps from natural compensation or perhaps because of the Prednisone, my left ear hearing had improved a little over the summer. I had years earlier given my left ear up for lost. It had gradually become so weak that by 2008, my brother, the audiology professor, had persuaded me to abandon my old in-ear hearing aid. He fitted me for a "BiCROS" hearing aid system. The aid I wore on my left had had both amplification and a tiny broadcasting device. Sound coming from my left would be picked up and relayed like a radio signal to a receiver on my right ear. The signal could be amplified, but my right ear was still so good at that point that amplification wasn't necessary.

The amazing thing about this system, Tim had told me, was that even though I would be hearing all the sound around me by way of my right ear, the brain—my brain—would adjust and make it possible to discern automatically where sounds were originating. I wouldn't have to worry about stepping into the path of a bus I thought was coming from the right when it was actually on my left.

He was correct. The BiCROS worked beautifully, at least until my good right ear died.

During my summer of drugs, however, the left ear had definitely made a comeback. I could hear water running in the sink. I could hear my own voice in my head. If Marty put her lips an inch or two from my ear and spoke slowly, I could understand simple questions like "Got...any...thoughts...about...dinner?"

I had the right-side half of my BiCROS system, the piece that could amplify, converted to fit my reborn left ear. It wasn't doing the right ear any good.

So, when Dr. Hoffmann asked which ear I wanted implanted, it was no contest. Now there are hybrid implants that allow a combination of digital stimulation and natural hearing. The implantation possible in 2010 would effectively "kill" the designated ear. If the implant doesn't work or you don't like how it sounds, too bad. The insertion does serious damage to the inner ear and is almost certainly irreparable. No way would I risk that little bit of left-ear hearing. With the implant stored away at night, my deafness would be total. I would not even be able to hear myself swallow. No way would I make this gamble. To this day, the first thing I do when I wake up in the morning is rub my hand across my outer left ear. I hear muffled, amorphous sound akin to the crumpling of paper. It is, metaphorically at least, music to my ear.

I told Dr. Hoffmann my left ear was off limits. Do the right thing.

Chapter 10

Masters of Disguise

O nly a few companies manufacture and market cochlear implants: Cochlear, MED-EL, and Advanced Bionics. Dr. Hoffmann, like all the Atlanta-area ear surgeons I surveyed, uses Cochlear exclusively. It's a company that originated in Australia but does the bulk of its business in the United States, with its headquarters in Denver. I was scheduled to be implanted with one of Cochlear's state-of-the-art Nucleus 5s in September.

Clear, frank, and thorough information about implants is not easy to come by. I am surely not the first prospective implantee to notice this, but I also would venture to say that my three decades in journalism, a field in which curiosity and skepticism are fundamental tools, made me acutely aware of it.

Dr. Hoffmann did show me a diagram of the Nucleus 5 and a sample. It's a spiny little thing that made me think of fossils of prehistoric fish I've seen on *Nature* or *NOVA*. The surgeon threads a fine wire festooned with twenty-two tiny transistors into the twisting chambers of the cochlea. The filament attaches to a chip, a teensy circuit board, that is placed just inside the skull, about an inch above the ear. The outer piece of the implant, the processor, looks and sits on the ear like a hearing aid, but in fact it's a powerful minicomputer that digitizes the sound waves it receives and transmits them to those microtransistors by way of a coil that attaches, like a refrigerator magnet, to the skull directly atop the metal disc inside your head.

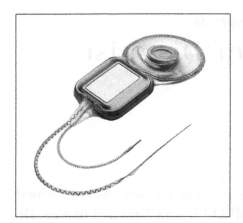 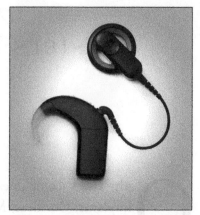

Courtesy of Cochlear Americas © 2020

Oddly, it was easier to get a glimpse of what would be inside my head than it was to get a clear idea of what the device was going to look like to other people. No doubt Cochlear Americas has research to prove that many potential implantees are anxious about becoming sideshow freaks or objects of derision. It's well known that thousands, perhaps millions, of people who would benefit greatly from hearing aids don't take advantage of the technology because, to some degree, they don't want to call attention to their disability. As I noted earlier, however, we, the hearing impaired, really can't afford such pride, such vanity. And it's disappointing that implant companies tend to cater to those worries rather than explode them.

The elaborate Cochlear promotional kit that Dr. Hoffmann gave me was as glossy and as short on hard information as a brochure for time-share condos on Maui. Photograph after photograph of satisfied implantees seemed carefully staged to demonstrate how easy it is to *hide* the device from view. The angle the person was shot from gave only a hint of the processor and coil, or the device was carefully covered by long hair.

What does one of these gizmos look like upside the head of a guy with a buzz cut or a shaved head? My hair was in fact medium long at the time, but I wanted to know what it was going to look like if I decided to try the Marine look.

I had to do Internet research to find a photo of an implant attached to someone with close-cropped hair. When I did, it was . . . interesting. The first one I saw looked like a charcoal-gray insect had attached itself to the guy's noggin. It looked to me like something that grew up to costar in *Aliens*, giving Sigourney Weaver's Ripley the fight of her life, or that would feed on my brain. It was kind of cool, actually, a potential conversation starter, assuming it indeed allowed me to converse.

I told myself the potential positives far outweighed the negatives. I repeated what was becoming my mantra:

Deaf be not proud. Deaf be not proud. Deaf be not proud.

Chapter 11
Goldberg Variations

We live in an age when surgeons can rebuild hearts; replace corneas, knees, and lungs; rewire brains; and equip amputees with race-track prosthetics, yet the inner ear remains challenging territory, a minuscule Marianas Trench inside your skull. It's complicated, delicate, and surrounded by hard, bony material that makes it difficult to reach without doing serious damage. As a cochlear audiologist once told me, the only way truly to have your ear examined and a problem diagnosed is for you to die so that a specialist could cut open your head and section the temporal bone. I did not want to know what was causing my hearing loss quite that badly.

Instead, I spent hours contemplating diagrams of the ear in the pages of books and on the screen of my computer.

In another essay published on www.likethedew.com, I noted that:

Going deaf tends to encourage that sort of thing. You want to know all you can about this sensory organ you until only recently had taken for granted.

Among other things, studying these drawings gave me new ideas about the nature of God. I came to believe that God is Rube Goldberg— or, at least, as the casting agents out the West Coast might say, a Rube Goldberg type.

For those possibly unfamiliar with his name and genius, Goldberg (1883–1970) was an author, an engineer, a sculptor and inventor. Most famously, he was a cartoonist who envisioned and drew comically complex devices that perform simple tasks in indirect, convoluted ways.

Keep Mr. Goldberg's work in mind as I briefly refresh your memory as to the construction and working of the intricate, delicate, sensitive, goofy apparatus we call the ear.

We gather and focus sound waves by way of the outer ear, outcroppings of cartilage and skin that grow on each side of our heads rather like mushrooms. I have the portabellas myself, but the model varies from person to person.

The outer ear, scientifically known as the pinna, directs the sound waves down a short tunnel, or canal, to the tympanic membrane, better known as the eardrum, which begins to vibrate from the pressure.

The vibration causes a chain reaction among the ossicles, three very tiny, closely connected bones on the other side of the eardrum, in the middle ear. The first bone, the malleus (hammer), moves from side to side like a lever, causing motion in the adjacent incus (anvil), which in turn jiggles the stapes (stirrup), which sends rippling waves through the fluid contained in the snail shell-shaped cochlea in the inner ear.

Tiny, hair-like cells inside the cochlea translate the wave motion into electrical impulses that travel along the auditory nerve to the brain. The brain decodes the impulses and makes it possible for us to discern whether what created the original vibration was a cat meowing or a politician barking or Eric Clapton playing slide guitar.

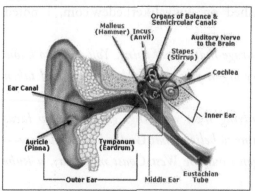

Courtesy of lyrichearing.com

Take a close look at the ear diagram included here. Now, take a close look at the classic Goldberg cartoon panel on the next page.

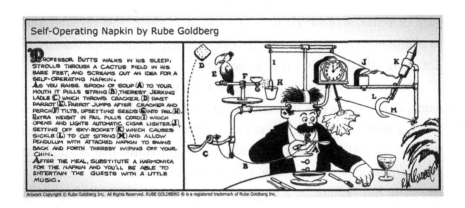

Self-Operating Napkin by Rube Goldberg

Isn't a contraption/process that involves a kitty's yowl, a drum, a hammer, an anvil, a stirrup and something that looks like it would make a nice home for a garden slug every bit as Goldberg-ian as a napkin-dabbing system that requires a clock, a scythe and a toucan?

Isn't it just as absurd? Isn't it, if anything, more miraculous?

*   *   *

There's more to it than this, of course. Rube took his time. Eons. The ears of mammals, ours included, are profound examples of evolutionary design, cumulative constructions that came together over a stretch of more than 250 million years.[5] Ears were the last paired organs to develop during evolution, and what we visualize when we say "ear," the visible outer ear, the pinna, developed last of all.

Primitive fish and, later, primitive amphibians "heard" by picking up vibrations through ground and water, much as salamanders do today. They detected vibration through their entire bodies, but mostly through the denser components, the bones. The complex, interactive parts of the ear—the ossicles, the tympanic membrane, and the coiled cochlea—developed slowly over time, as conditions and needs changed. Air doesn't conduct vibration as well as soil and

5   Geoffrey A. Manley, "Aural History," *The Scientist*, Sept. 1, 2015, https://www.the-scientist.com/features/aural-history-34918.

rock or water, so animals that spent most of their time on land and in the open had to adapt, to develop keener, more subtle means of detecting vibrations in order to survive.

Our ears aren't the best in the animal world, but they're not the worst, either. Ours can differentiate up to four hundred thousand different sounds. They can process more impressions than our eyes, about fifty per second.[6] On first impulse, you might think that if surgeons can transplant hearts, lending a deaf person an ear would be a relative snap. But no, not by a long shot. Surgical techniques for replacing the stapes (stirrup) have been around for more than four decades, with a near-imperishable polymer prosthesis now replacing the earlier silver replacement part. But the inner ear, in which most causes of deafness originate, is a surgical challenge far more daunting than connecting an artificial heart or reattaching a severed limb.

"First of all, the inner ear is a tiny, pea-sized organ located within the temporal bone, one of the hardest bones in the body," my brother, Dr. J. Timothy Holston, told me. He's a longtime professor at the University of South Alabama, now retired, and past president of the Alabama Academy of Audiology.

"Accessibility is not easy," he further explained. "Second, the inner ear is very complex—they don't call it the 'labyrinth' for nothing. You have two different fluids in the inner ear, both of which have different electrical polarities that have to remain balanced. Also, the interconnections between the sensory hair cells (two kinds, inner and outer, both of which have different functions) and the nerve endings at their base are quite complex."

Dr. William Slattery, a surgeon and researcher at the House Institute in Los Angeles, told me that while it would be wonderful to transplant cochleas, it's beyond our surgical capabilities now. Large organs like the heart and liver, while complex, provide much

6 "How the Hearing Works," Hear the World Foundation, accessed May 21, 2019, https://www.hear-the-world.com/en/knowledge/hearing/how-hearing-works.

simpler functions. Not only is the cochlea smaller than a jelly bean, but its functions are dramatically more diverse and complicated than those of the larger organs.

"There are fifteen thousand hair cells that each respond to different frequencies [and they're] packed within the area the size of a pea," Slattery said. "And this is only one type of cell. In addition to this, there are supporting cells, there are fluid regulation cells. It is truly a quite complex organization that requires all of these mechanisms to be working together and in sync.

"Transplanting a cochlea would then require the nerves to all function properly. It is kind of like taking a piano of fifteen thousand keys and trying to transplant that with input of all these different frequencies."

Cochlear implants continue to be refined. New models developed by Cochlear Limited and MED-EL are hybrids—part implant, part hearing aid. They're primarily for people who have better hearing in the low frequencies but drop to a severe/profound deficit in the mid-to-high frequencies. "The hearing aid part of the device works for the lows, while the implant part stimulates the mid-highs, where the aid is not effective," Tim said.

Scientists also have developed a prototype for a "bionic cochlea" that mimics the function of the inner ear. "The problem would be getting something like that to a size that would approximate the tiny inner ear and getting it in via the temporal bone," Tim said. "If this ever came to fruition, I think it would have to be something external that would perform the function of the cochlea."

Researchers are continuing to experiment with chemical and drug therapies, including treatments that would regenerate hair cells. "This has been much more difficult than initially proposed," Slattery said. "Much of this work started in 1995. As you can see, it is now twenty years later and we still do not have treatments for this type of hair cell loss."

We have known since the late 1980s that the ears of young chickens are able to regrow dead hair cells and regain lost hearing.[7] A mammal with similar capability has yet to be discovered, but scientists remain intrigued by the possibility that a way to induce hair-cell regrowth in humans may be found. A research project at Massachusetts Eye and Ear is perhaps a preview: scientists have had some success restoring the damaged hearing of test mice with a drug that was developed to treat Alzheimer's.[8]

"Research on regenerating hair cells is promising and perhaps closer to coming to fruition that we might think," Dr. Holston said. "The primary avenues of study are in genetic modification of supporting cells that exist around the hair cells into actual hair cells. The other is using embryonic stem cells that may have a propensity to develop into hair cells and placing them with supporting cells with the hope that they will develop into hair cells. Again, the problem is that, once you've developed the hair cells, will they make the complex re-connections with the underlying nerve fibers and would there be any relearning process, as you go through with a cochlear implant."

Slatttery said the major focus of treating hearing loss has become "trying to prevent further loss of hearing. The goal is to try and stabilize patients when they are first experiencing some kind of hearing loss."

A Paul McCartney song comes to mind, the bittersweet "Tug of War." Macca ruefully acknowledges that revelations and discoveries about science and life, inevitable though they may be in the future, won't happen while he's still drawing breath and dreaming up melodies.

---

7   "Do You Hear What I Hear: All About Chicken Hearing," *Fresh Eggs Daily,* September, 2016, https://www.fresheggsdaily.com/2016/09/do-you-hear-what-i-hear-all-about.html.

8   Jon Hamilton, "Alzheimer's Drug Dials Back Deafness in Mice," National Public Radio, January 9, 2013, https://www.npr.org/sections/health-shots/2013/01/09/168960377/mice-dial-back-deafness-with-alzheimers-drug.

Chapter 12

Drill, Baby, Drill

M y implantation surgery was set for September 27 at Atlanta's Piedmont Hospital. Every professional with whom Marty and I consulted, including Dr. Hoffmann and my brother, Tim, said that given my age, excellent overall health, high educational level, work ethic, and the recency of my hearing loss, the odds of a favorable outcome were very good. Education, I was told, indicated that I would have a larger vocabulary from which to identify words I'd be hearing in a new, digitized form. My work history predicted diligence, while the newness of my hearing loss meant that I, unlike a lifelong or longtime deaf person getting an implant, would not be starting from ground zero.

Life, meanwhile, had thrown us another curve. In August, Marty had found a lump in her right breast. A biopsy determined that it was cancerous. Her surgery, a lumpectomy, was scheduled for less than a week after mine. She had been the proverbial saint during the early months of my hearing loss, diligently making and taking phone calls I could not, scheduling me for medical appointments and haircuts, painstakingly writing down her thoughts on a steno pad so we could "converse," nagging me about practicing sign language, and endlessly repeating words and phrases I didn't understand.

I had heard it said, as a bitter joke, that nothing undermines a good marriage worse than the death of a child or a kitchen remodeling. To that short list I would add sudden deafness.

Marty's patience withered after her cancer diagnosis. She was frightened and frantic, suddenly resentful of the time and effort I required. For as long as I had known her, she had had an acute sense of life slipping away. One of her songs, "Sand," begins, "There is only so much sand/In the hourglass/In the hourglass." Another, "Big Brass Ring," has a bridge that includes the lines "You never know when this life/Is going to end/Stop putting your todays off until tomorrow."

Now she was on a tear, a binge, getting out of bed in the middle of the night, rearranging the furniture almost daily, dragging old photos and half-finished lyrics out of boxes in closets and leaving a trail of clutter like Pigpen in the *Peanuts* comic strip.

I was already on edge. Now I was alarmed and discombobulated. I worried that she might be losing her mind. I expressed my fears to my stepdaughter, Downie, who shared the conversation with her mom. Marty sent me a stinging email—at that point the surest way to communicate with me—and laid out her frustration and anger.

"I realize that you've had something very traumatic happen to you in the past seven months," she said. "So have I.

"I need to write," she continued. "I need time to myself. I need not to have anyone else insist that their needs are greater. Part of why my illness came to light (belatedly) is because I didn't have time to find the lump. We've been super-focused on you. We need to focus on me. Or I need to focus on me. I can't tell you how angry I am. I feel taken advantage of and taken for granted, the whole nine yards."

It was a kick in the head. Through six increasingly frustrating months, I had continued to go to work at the Peabodys and bring home a paycheck. I did most of the cooking, most of the yard-work, and more than my fair share of housework (Marty was raised in a Nebraska house that looks like a thrift store tossed by Drug Enforcement Agency operatives and has no problem with clutter). Friends and colleagues had praised me for the grace and humor with which they believed I was dealing with my deafness, and I was only too happy to agree with them. But none of them, I finally realized, had to be around me twelve or fourteen waking hours a day. None of them comprehended what it was like for Marty to have to repeat the simplest comments and requests again and again. None of them knew what it was like to have a partner who couldn't listen, not deeply and fully anyway, or who was too consumed with anxiety and the difficulty of everyday activities to be truly empathetic. But that was me. Unintentionally or not, that was me.

As my surgery date approached, we aired out our differences. We had some marriage counseling sessions with a therapist we found insightful, compassionate, and frank. We went bird-watching, one of Marty's favorite pastimes, at lakes and swamps where *not* talking was essential. We went dancing—I could feel deep bass notes even if I couldn't hear them, and I could watch Marty's movements for cues. We got to what seemed like a better place.

Marty made a barber shop appointment for me. I got my hair buzzed. Then, at home, I shaved my head completely, figuring most of my hair would go at the pre-op anyway. I hadn't had short-short hair since I was a little kid. I wanted to be proactive, make a game of it, and see what I looked like in Howie Mandel mode. I fantasized about trying out for the Yul Brynner role in a community theater production of *The King and I* once my hearing was restored. Etcetera, etcetera, etcetera.

We decided that we should get a motel room in Atlanta for the Sunday night before my Monday morning surgery. Under perfect circumstances, it would be an hour-and-a-half drive from Athens to the hospital. We didn't want to risk a delay caused by workday traffic, let alone drive in it. We planned to head for Atlanta Sunday afternoon, check in to the motel, take a dip in the pool, and have a leisurely dinner someplace cool. And I, at least, was thinking we would have time for some motel romance, a last tryst in case I didn't wake up from the anesthesia.

The best laid plans of laboratory mice and men . . .

We were late getting on the road to Atlanta. Like, two hours late. When we were on I-85, well inside the sprawling city's boundaries, we realized we had left the motel reservation, including its address, at home. When Marty attempted to call the motel on her cell phone, hoping for guidance, she discovered she could only get a national switchboard. The operator on duty could find no trace of our reservation at any of the chain's outlets in greater Atlanta. Marty had to make a new reservation and, because we were largely ignorant of Atlanta's layout, had to guess which one was closest to the hospital. The operator, who was in Ohio or maybe India, was no help.

We eventually found ourselves checking into a slightly sooty franchise built cheek to jowl with a freeway cloverleaf seventeen miles from the hospital. I could not hear the ceaseless whoosh of cars. Marty could. We got no pool time. After a tense cruising of the nearby strip malls, we ended up eating dinner at about 9:30 p.m. at a fast-food restaurant. Back at the motel, we collapsed into bed so exhausted we were barely able to undress.

Wake-up time—4:30 a.m.—came painfully early for both of us. At least I had the comfort of knowing I would soon be getting anesthesia.

I wasn't especially nervous. I hadn't had surgery since I had my tonsils removed in my Mississippi hometown when I was eight. It left no traumatic memories. I recall somebody putting a mask over my face, the smell of a chemical, and the words "Count backwards from ten." I only got as far as eight before a peaceful pitch-blackness enveloped me. And afterward, when I awoke, I got ice cream. I was counting on more of the same.

It was strange to be inside a hospital so early in the day. With few people around, it's sort of comforting, as if all its staff and machinery were there just for you. On the other hand, the handful of nonstaff people in the waiting room looked tired, sad, worried, even doomed. It occurred to me that I probably looked the same way to them. I was glad when we were summoned to pre-op.

I've read all sorts of horror stories about surgical patients picking up staph infections and such at hospitals. My father-in-law, Don Winkler, had a terrible experience with staph following bypass surgery at a hospital in Nebraska. I'm not sure how this kind of thing can happen if the average hospital is kept as cold as Piedmont. I felt fully refrigerated. I figured bacteria would go into hibernation. I put on my gown and no-slip socks, bagged up my belongings, and crawled under the covers. A nurse took my vitals and started a drip to relax me in advance of the anesthesia. Dr. Hoffmann dropped by to reassure me. She also pulled a magic marker from her pocket and drew an arrow on my right cheek pointing to my right ear. I was happy for the precaution but a little dismayed by the need for it.

I was alert, if not exactly wide awake, when Marty kissed me and mouthed, "I love you." An orderly rolled me into the operating room. On my back, I could see lots of chrome and glaring lights. I flashed on the old *Twilight Zone* episode in which the doctors and nurses hovering over a surgical patient turn out to have faces like pigs. I was able to watch the silent ballet of masked women and men until I faded blissfully into deep, dark, dreamless sleep.

What happened between then and my groggy awakening I got secondhand, of course.

First, Dr. Hoffmann took a scalpel and cut along the back of my pinna, my outer ear, and folded it forward and out of the way like the page of a calendar. Then, using a high-speed, diamond-bit drill,

Dr. Hoffmann bored through my skull an inch above my outer ear. Then she tunneled through the mastoid bone toward my cochlea, about an inch and a half away. What might seem like the obvious route—directly through the ear canal—is not an option. It's too open. There's nothing to which the implant wire's electrode array can be attached. Plus, going through the ear canal would entail puncturing the eardrum, thus leaving the middle ear exposed to dust, gnats, and water.

Dr. Hoffmann confided later that she had initially had difficulty finding my cochlea. All our cochlea are well protected by bone and thus hard to get at, but mine apparently was better hidden than most. She told Marty she was on the verge of calling another ear surgeon on her cell to get some advice when she finally spied the little nautilus, no bigger than a bean. I had visions of her being a contestant on *Who Wants to Be a Millionaire* and being obliged to use up one of her "lifeline" calls—in order to stay in the game.

When she did locate my cochlea, it was problematic. She said she "met with resistance," rather like what happens when you snake out a kitchen drain pipe and meet with a tricky bend. She said she wasn't sure if she'd gotten the electrode array completely into my cochlea but that, otherwise, the surgery had gone smoothly. She had threaded the array into the cochlea—I imagined it as rather like probing a crawdad hole with a blade of grass, as I had done as a country child—and secured its dime-sized head, a computer chip, in the cavity she had drilled, now reupholstered with my skin.

Would it work, would it give me back some useful hearing capacity? I would find out in a month. It can take that long for the incision to heal and for the tissue to start growing around the new "bionic" parts. Attaching the exterior processor, a mated magnet, might pull the electrode array out of line. The only certainty at this moment was that I would never hear naturally with my right ear again. No matter which medical breakthroughs lie ahead, no serum or stimuli would revive my cochlea. Implantation almost always equals destruction. I was sure my right ear was DOI (dead on implantation).

Foggy and wobbly, with a white gauze pad like one of Madonna's notorious breastplates taped over my right ear, I was with Marty in her little Nissan Sentra heading back to Athens by 3 p.m. That's 3 p.m. of the same day. The hole in the head notwithstanding, a cochlear implantation is more often than not an outpatient surgery.

What I wanted most in the world was to get home and climb into bed with the blinds down and the curtains pulled. What Marty wanted most in the world was to get home and climb into bed with the blinds down and the curtains pulled. Like me, she had had virtually no sleep the night before. Unlike me, she hadn't spent three hours that morning in chemically induced oblivion. I was groggy. She, though I didn't fully appreciate it at the time, was brain burned.

The timing of my hospital discharge couldn't have been poorer. From our house in Athens to Piedmont Hospital is an hour-and-a-half drive between midnight and 5 a.m. Any other time of day, that's the minimum you can expect. We headed out as the city's infamous rush hour was starting—five or six lanes of traffic in each direction, cars and trucks blasting along at sixty-five to seventy miles per hour, most of them tailgating. Marty made it down I-285, the Atlanta Bypass, and north up I-85 past Jimmy Carter Boulevard to the exit for Athens, Georgia, 316, without getting bashed. But a couple of miles east of 85, she suddenly pulled off the highway to a side road and then an empty parking lot.

I was baffled. "What are you doing?"

"Have to sleep," she mouthed.

"We're only about thirty-five minutes from home," I said. "The painkillers are starting to wear off. I need to get home, take another pill, and lie down."

She pulled out her steno pad. "If I don't sleep a little, we will never make it home," she wrote. And with that, she lowered the windows slightly, turned off the engine, ratcheted back her seat, and closed her eyes. I tried to lean my head against the window, letting the fat bandage function like an airline pillow, and listened to the newly aggravated sounds in my head. It sounded like Gamelan, the music of Bali, all gongs and bells and, to my Western ears, dissonance.

Chapter 13

Helplessly Hoping

Two days after my surgery, one of Marty's older sisters, Margaret, a retired nurse, flew in from Texas to help out. Two days after that, Marty had a malignant mass removed from her right breast, along with lymph nodes for testing, at Athens Regional.

Margaret had volunteered to cook for us and keep the house straight while Marty and I recovered, but what we really needed her for was her ears. We desperately needed an intermediary who could understand what the doctors and nurses said and ask them questions. We needed someone who could take phone calls when Marty was asleep.

We were aware that there were special telephones on the market that use voice-recognition technology to translate a caller's words into text and display them on a screen. But acquiring gadgets of that sort seemed premature, not to mention kind of defeatist. So what if I was conversationally useless at the moment? I was on the brink of a breakthrough; I was going to hear.

My recovery, physically at least, was speedy. I'd had root canals that left me more drained. I was up and around in a couple of days, moving slow but definitely moving. Marty's lumpectomy took a harder toll. The surgeon had removed the lump from her breast and some of the lymph nodes under her right arm. Beneath the bandages wrapped tightly around her chest and back, she was badly bruised. She was in pain, feverish, frightened, and angry. Frightened because, well, who wouldn't be? And she was doubly sensitive to the possibilities because another of her sisters, Amy, was battling a form of cancer for which there was no known cure. She was angry because she had in the previous year made some serious headway in her musical ambitions, releasing *Under Your Heart,* a CD of her songs (and ours), and getting chosen to perform live at Athfest, the city's annual summer music festival, and to be included on its sampler CD. And here she was with a husband with an energy-draining illness and a potentially life-threatening malady of her own. Weeks of radiation therapy awaited her, side effects unknown.

The first week was like living a John Cassavetes movie—*A Man and Woman Under the Influence.* I had never felt more isolated or helpless. My left ear was good enough for only the simplest phrases, spoken just an inch away. Activation of my implant was weeks away, leaving me with no hearing in my right ear, just growing tinnitus. I could read. I could try to watch TV with captions. I could email. But meaningful conversation was so difficult, it scarcely seemed worth the exertion. I alternated between depression and mild hysteria.

Mild is how it seemed to me. Marty believed I was overreacting to the slightest provocations, from the clutter in the house to her mood swings. I thought she was losing touch with reality. Margaret refereed as best she could. She knew her sister; she had helped raise her. She knew me only from an hour here and there at family reunions and thus had no way of knowing if my behavior was better or worse than usual.

On Saturday, the day after her surgery, Marty felt surprising well and decided she wanted to show Margaret something of Athens besides a hospital. She had Margaret drive her to Athens's Memorial Park, where we often go to walk around the big pond, feed the turtles and ducks, and tour the small zoo of native-to-Georgia rescue animals. Margaret thought she was attempting to do too much too soon, but Marty insisted. She craves the outdoors.

All was well, or so we thought. She awakened on Sunday morning with a fever and having what she said felt like an asthma attack. She was panicking; I couldn't think straight. Margaret took over. "There's a type of pneumonia that's specific to hospitals," she said. "We're going to the ER."

At St. Mary's Hospital's emergency room, a doctor checked her breathing, prescribed an antibiotic, and chastised her for ignoring her surgeon's order to take it slow and easy. This time, with Margaret taking on the role of tough cop, she listened.

To keep herself busy while resting, Marty planned a party by phone and text. October 10 was Downie's birthday and, as it happened, Margaret's, too. Marty managed to keep both in the dark by telling Downie it was a surprise for Margaret and vice versa. The venue she picked was a Vietnamese cafe where Downie worked part-time. The owners were only too happy to be in on the plot. Marty invited a half-dozen friends of ours and Downie's and told them to be at the restaurant at 6 p.m.

That Friday afternoon, Marty, Downie, and Margaret headed to a nearby nail salon for a "girls" outing, leaving me by myself at the house. As party time approached and they hadn't returned, I texted Marty. She texted back that the manis and pedis were taking longer than expected and that I should go on to the restaurant by myself. They'd meet me there.

I was annoyed. I felt as though I had a diving bubble or space helmet hermetically sealed over my head. What was I supposed to do at the restaurant? Greet the guests with notes on a pad? I got in my car, felt rather than heard the engine catch, and drove to the restaurant. Some of the guests were already there, waiting to go, "Surprise!" Instead they said, "Where's Downie? Where's Marty?" I watched their mouths, figured out the words, pulled out a steno pad, and wrote, "Getting nails done. Running late."

They gave me quizzical looks, asked me how I was doing— my head was still bandaged—and soon became immersed in conversation among themselves. I listened to the white noise, did my best to smile when someone looked at me, and watched my watch. I was anxious and getting angrier by the minute. Now would be a good time for space aliens to abduct me, I thought. Just shoot down a beam and vacuum me right up into the mother ship.

When Marty and the birthday girls sashayed in merrily almost an hour late, I got up and gave each a hug and a kiss on the cheek. A splendid time was apparently had by all. I thought the party would never end.

The day after we drove Margaret to the airport in Atlanta, Marty wrote on a steno pad, "I think you ought to go to Laurel to see Nell." Nell is Nell Damon, my late mother's only sister and one of my few surviving relatives of that generation. She and my mom had sold their respective houses and bought another one together when I was in my early twenties, and they had remained roommates until my mom's death in 2003.

My first reaction upon reading Marty's note was "You've got to be kidding." Laurel was more than seven hours away, and she expected me to jump in the car and drive there by myself. I was uneasy just driving to my job on the university campus, less than three miles from home.

I was a little surprised I was actually allowed to drive. Marty had taken to referring to me as "legally deaf" when she made medical-related phone calls for me; plus, it gave her a quick, easy out when telemarketers called for me. "I'm sorry, but Mr. Holston is *legally deaf.*"

There's no such designation in the law. Legally blind, yes. That means you can see a little something but not nearly enough to be allowed behind the wheel of a car. But legally deaf, no. You can still get a driver's license and chauffeur yourself around solo even though you can't hear a fast-approaching ambulance's siren or another

motorist's honking horn. To compensate, you have to constantly dart your eyes from mirror to mirror, pay attention like you haven't since you were getting your learner's permit, anticipate, anticipate, anticipate, grit your teeth, and pray.

On the long drive to southeast Mississippi, there would be all that and more. I couldn't buy chips and a Coke at a convenience store without having the clerk write the amount on a pad. If I got stopped by the cops, they might mistake me in my uncertainty for a drunk. If had car trouble, my AAA card would be useless. I couldn't make the call. I didn't just dread the trip, I was two steps shy of panic.

But Marty was adamant. She needed space. She needed time alone. She said she couldn't continue to deal with my deafness while she was dealing with postsurgical pain and thinking ahead to the recommended radiation therapy. She wanted me out of the house. She phoned my aunt and said, "Hey, guess what. Noel's coming to see you." Or so she wrote on the pad a little later.

I had made the drive from Athens to Laurel by myself a dozen times when I was on a fellowship at the University of Georgia in the mid-1990s. I knew the Athens to Atlanta to Birmingham to Tuscaloosa to Meridian to Laurel route well. But on those trips, I had had radio news and CDs to keep me alert and awake. I had a cache of preferred driving music—the B-52's, Tom Petty, Alison Krauss, an anthology of Big Band-era classics featuring the likes of Duke Ellington, Benny Goodman, and Fletcher Henderson. Like Bobby McGee, I rode a song of wind across Alabama to my hometown. But for this trip, I would have no outside aural stimulation, just nerves, strong coffee, and all the bone-conducted head-noise I could generate.

Marty kissed me good-bye. It felt more like she was kissing me off. As I drove up the hill through our neighborhood to the highway that leads to Atlanta, I was uncertain, befuddled, and embarrassed. And pissed. I wanted to say, "If you need space so badly, why don't you jump in *your* car and go somewhere?" But she was even less fit to travel than I, so I gave our old Nissan a little more gas and headed west. I could barely hear the engine or the tires on the pavement. I wondered if this was what space travel "sounded" like.

By the time I got past the auto dealerships and furniture stores on Athens's fringe and turned onto Hwy 316, I was already getting anxious about simply getting around Atlanta, sixty minutes away. After living on Long Island and negotiating the notorious LI Expressway, I thought I would be comfortable driving anywhere. But Atlanta is insane. To get around it and on the road to Birmingham, you have to do fourteen miles on I-85 and another twenty on the 285 Bypass, both five lanes wide and teeming from early, early morning until late at night with cars, pickups, and semis going seventy miles per hour or more. I hated driving in Atlanta under the best of circumstances.

Interstate 85 was the raceway I expected. Both hands on the wheel, white-knuckled, I picked a right-side lane and stayed there, my eyes flitting constantly from rear-view to side mirrors to survey speeding Beamers and roaring trucks that made no sound for me beyond white noise. When I finally got to the exit for I-20 west of Atlanta, I took a deep breath and said a prayer of thanks. At the first rest area, I parked and walked to one of the concrete picnic tables. I climbed on the slab, lay down on my back, and closed my eyes. "Telstar" played on the phantom CD player in my head, oddly comforting, as though I were in orbit.

To make sure I stayed awake the rest of the seven-and-a-half-hour drive, I talked to myself and sang old favorites—"You've Lost That Loving Feeling" seemed particularly appropriate, as did "Honky Tonk Women." I sang a cappella, masochistically off-key, and as loud as I could so that I could sort of hear myself by bone conduction. I took special note of the scenery. The stretch of interstate east of Birmingham is especially gorgeous, the exposed granite walls rising on either side looking not so much blasted as sculpted, chiseled by giants. I had always noticed it before. It's impossible not to notice. But this time I really looked, really savored. It was a habit, I said to myself, that I needed to develop.

My Aunt Nell greeted me at the front door of her red-brick house with a warm smile and a drawled greeting I could not hear. She already had a note pad out on the dining room table. The first question she wrote was "Do you want pecan pie, chess pie, or pound cake?" I opted for some of each. It was good to be home and good to be babied a bit.

For three days, I did little beyond read magazines and let Nell stuff me with fried chicken, turnip greens, and twice-baked potatoes. At night, we watched old movies my late mom had videotaped off Turner Classics—*An Affair to Remember, Casablanca, Gaslight*—or played Scrabble like we used to do when my brother and I were kids.

I went grocery shopping with her wearing a ski cap for which it was much too warm. Better that the customers at Piggly Wiggly glance at the cap, though, than gawk at the strip above my ear that still made it look like someone had trimmed my hair with a blowtorch. I begged off on joining Nell for church on Sunday at First Methodist. I later caught myself humming "Eleanor Rigby," triggered by memory of the line about a sermon falling on deaf ears.

On Monday, I headed back to Athens, once again keeping myself awake with a thermos of coffee and loud singing. Marty and I hadn't spoken in days. Phoning wasn't an option. Nell called her to tell her I was on my way.

When I got home, Marty was in a conciliatory mood. She greeted me with a kiss at the door and proudly led me to the dining room, where she was setting out a pot roast dinner. All I could see was that the house was a mess, the table cleared just enough to put down place mats, the kitchen sink filled with pots and dishes, and the counter tops strewn with junk mail and rocks she had collected from the creek behind our house. The usual clutter. I didn't complain, but annoyance was written all over my face. We ate in silence, both of us fuming, not even bothering to scribble notes on a pad. We slept on opposite edges of the bed.

The next morning, she asked me to walk outside with her. She led me down our sloping driveway to the tuck-under garage and pointed up to the expanse of stucco above the double-wide door. My mouth fell open. On the wall, in purple and day-glow green spray paint, she had outlined the abstract figure of a woman, about four feet by four, in a large, billowing skirt. Waves of wiggly green and purple stripes pulsed out from both sides.

"We've talked about having a mural done for years," she mouthed. "So . . ."

I couldn't think of anything to say. Leastways, nothing that wasn't a string of expletives I would regret. Sure, we had talked about a mural. There was an antique shop near downtown that had a mural, a portrait of a bed of bright flowers, on a side wall. We'd talked about hiring one of our neighbors, a visual artist who had muralized the concrete fence around her patio, to do something similar for us. But this—to me, in my shock—just looked like graffiti, like Marty had taken it upon herself to deface our house.

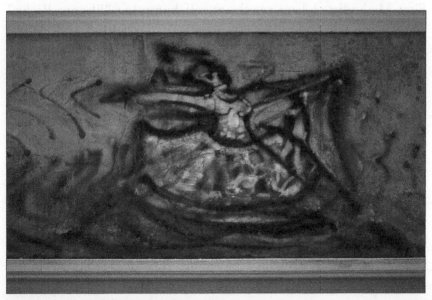

I hiked up the driveway, got into my car, and drove off. I went to a church parking lot up the hill and walked off—and cursed off—my anger.

Luckily, we had a counseling session scheduled two days later. With our therapist mediating, I expressed my dismay that Marty would mark up the side of our house without consulting me. She explained that the "Dancing Lady," as she had titled her day-glow fresco, was not just another of her kooky decorating impulses like hanging old computer discs on strings from tree limbs or lining flower beds with stray hubcaps. It was a way of reclaiming her body after her cancer surgery.

Our therapist reminded us what different people we are in many ways—deliberative vs. spontaneous, Dr. Fickle vs. Ms. In Stride—but that we share so many more important values. She reminded us that we were each undergoing a life-changing experience that, by itself, would strain a marriage. This was a double whammy. She encouraged Marty to be more cognizant of the possible impact of her impulses and encouraged me to work on my ability to go with the flow.

When we got home—we'd gone to counseling in separate cars—I walked down the driveway and looked at the Dancing Lady. Really looked. Studied the motion suggested by the skirt and the radiating lines. It was actually pretty good.

Chapter 14

We'll Remember Always, Activation Day

On the evening of my October 26 implant activation, I sent an email to my sons in Minneapolis and copied a few friends, relatives, and in-laws. I wrote:

The audiologist programmed and activated my implant this afternoon. It was exciting, surprising and, truth be told, kind of daunting. Nothing I'd read really prepared me for what this is going to be like—a long, slow, learning experience.

I'm a newborn baby, hearing-wise. I have to re-learn how everything sounds.

Here's why (short, oversimplified version): We learn how the world sounds as infants by gradually associating naturally created electrical impulses with thousands of things: words, the bark of a dog, the rattle and pop of an ice maker, the scratch of a match on a box. I am now getting those electrical impulses artificially from my sound processor (hearing aid-like ear piece). They aren't the same impulses I got with a healthy cochlea, but my brain will eventually match the impulses to words, sounds, etc. It will take time and practice, practice, practice.

Right now, I can't identify any specific sound with my "bionic" ear. I hear a kind of tinkling that reminds me of a tiny, wind-up music box. It's like Tinkerbell is flitting about inside my ear. The encouraging thing is that the tinklings have different tones, patterns, and cadences that I can clearly discern even though I don't know what they say/mean just yet.

My job for the next week, before I go back to see the audiologist for more programming, is to feed my brain information so it can make new associations. I am supposed to not only watch and listen closely to people talking to me but to make note of how the slamming of a door "sounds" to my new ear—and how my car sounds when I start it and how the blinkers sound. I also have to condition my ear, which hasn't heard much in months, to accommodate more and louder sounds. I will work my way up in volume.

Amber Rolfes, a clinical audiologist at Piedmont ENT, could only activate a portion of the little electrodes now arrayed in my cochlea, lest the auditory nerve be overwhelmed. Every time she activates more electrodes, the range of what I will be able to hear will increase.

She said this is going to take time and lots of concentration and patience on my part. But she assured me I would eventually be hearing more and better than I have heard in a long, long time—meaning well before my hearing got truly bad. Unlike blindness, deafness can sneak up on you without you even noticing what you lost.

So, yippee yi yay! I am glad to be getting started and am hoping for the best.

One little drawback: I will be deafer than usual for a while. The hearing aid I've been using in my left ear, the one that still has some residual hearing, has been declared off limits. I've been told not to use it for six months, so that my right ear won't have a crutch.

So, that's it for now.

Well, one other thing: I had no clue, despite all that I read, that the cochlear implant business would be so complicated. My Cochlear Nucleus 5 kit—full of accessories, manuals, educational CDs, battery chargers, you name it—is the size of a carry-on suitcase. There's even a cord I will be able to plug into a stereo or iPod and relay music directly into my head. Gives a whole new meaning to the term "wired for sound," eh?

Love to you all and thank you for your concern.
Be hearing you soon.
Dad/Noel

*   *   *

There's more to it than that. We started the day with a drive from Athens to Piedmont Medical, a steel-gray high-rise in Buckhead that's home to Dr. Hoffmann's practice. The drive is ninety minutes on the best, free-flowing traffic day. We gave ourselves an extra half hour to be on the safe side and needed every extra minute. Marty had to drop me off and go look for parking while I made my way upstairs.

My appointment was with Ms. Rolfes, a relative newcomer to cochlear audiology and a new mom. She had in fact missed my surgery because she had been on leave, giving birth. She had in fact been on leave, giving birth, when Dr. Hoffmann was giving me my bionic ear.

One of the first things I noticed in her little office was a framed poster provided by Siemens, a hearing-aid manufacturer: intricate pen-and-ink renderings of antique hearing devices, including the sort of ear horns I associate with ancient, bearded men in rocking chairs on the porches of Confederate veterans' homes. I think the poster was there to convey the subtle message that this, not so long ago, could have been *your* fate.

Amber opened my Nucleus 5 kit, a multilayered suitcase that resembled an extra-extra-large Whitman's Sampler, with individually boxed processors, coils, magnets, a remote control, batteries, chargers, and ear clips instead of assorted chocolates. She held up one of my processors. It was gun-metal gray, the color chosen in advance by me to blend in with my salt-and-pepper hair. No bigger than a jalapeño, this compact computer would sit atop my right ear, lightly, I soon discovered; the wire, the "coil," extended from the back of it. The dime-sized magnet at the other end would stick to the chip just inside my skull. Sounds detected by the processor would be relayed through the coil and fire the tiny electrodes deep in my cochlea.

Amber emphasized that the processor is in no way a hearing aid. It would not amplify sound. Rather, it would convert the sounds it detects into digital signals to which the electrodes on the wire would respond. It would *approximate* sound.

She reminded me that my left-ear hearing aid was off limits for a month. To cheat, she said, would only impede the process of my brain adapting to the new, digitized way of hearing. She also made a prediction that made my heart leap.

"In a few months, you probably won't even want to bother with the hearing aid," she said. "You will be hearing so much with your implant, you won't think it's necessary."

She was getting a wee bit ahead of herself. Before she could activate my implant, she had to calibrate it. She attached a thin, three-foot cable to her laptop and the other end to my processor. I sat the earpiece on my ear and moved the magnet across my skull until I felt it adhere. It made no sound. I could only feel a light, firm suction.

For the next half hour, though it seemed longer, I heard—well, sort of heard/sort of felt—a succession of beeps inside my head. The beeps would start faintly, grow steadily stronger, then fade again. There would be a slight pause, and then the beep, rising then falling in intensity, would repeat. What Amber was doing was testing the electrodes in the array one by one, ensuring each was functioning and determining how much stimulation I could take at each point. It wasn't a purely passive experience for me. At each point, I had to tell Amber when she reached the limit of my comfort level. The last thing we wanted was to activate the processor and have a blast of digital sound like a Jimmy Page power chord in my cranium.

The rock analogy is apt. Programming a processor—"mapping" as it's known—is very much like sound checks I've participated in when I was singing with Marty. You're standing on the stage with a row of monitors at your feet. The sound person is standing before a board full of levers and dials on the other side of the club or up on the balcony. Like a cochlear audiologist, the sound person is trying to give you a mix you want—a bit more bass, a little less reverb, bring up the volume a notch. He or she can't hear what you hear. The sound person, or the audiologist, can only take in your verbal feedback and try to translate it into sound you approve, or at least can live with.

The big reveal was only minutes away. I had been told the voices I would hear with the implant might sound like Mickey Mouse's. That's apparently what many implantees have reported. I've also read that what I heard might remind me of Stephen Hawking, the astrophysicist, speaking through his voice box. And I had more or less concluded, from a listen during one of my steroid-spiked upswings, that what I was going to hear initially might sound like performance artist-turned-pop star Laurie Anderson using her vocoder, on tunes like "O Superman."

I was OK with that. Initially at least, I would be happy with a return of basic function. I would worry about fidelity later.

With Marty sitting across from me—her fingers crossed, as were mine—Amber turned me on.

It was as if . . . as if . . . as if I had just flipped on an old, nondigital radio and landed somewhere between signals. There was only static. White noise. Shzzzzzzzzzzzzzzzzzzzzzzzzzzzz.

Where's Mickey Mouse? I wondered. *Where's Minnie Mouse? Any mouse?*

"Somebody say something," I said. What I heard in my head was "shzzzzzbizz sss sssstim."

I saw Marty's lips moving. I heard "Shzzzzzz chzzzzzzt tssss chvzzzzr." I had no idea what the words were, but, on the plus side, I knew she was indeed speaking words. I could detect cadence, rhythm. I could tell some of the indecipherable words were longer than others.

There was nothing more Amber could do at our session. She wrote on a pad that I needed to give my brain time to begin making sense of the approximated sounds the processor was delivering. Like a baby who gradually differentiates thousands and thousands of variants in what at first seems a storm of furious, inescapable sound, I would sort it out. And because I was an adult who has spent years hearing, I would do it faster.

"It will get better," she said, looking straight at me and pantomiming the words.

Still, she couldn't hide that she was disappointed. Marty and I were, too. Our drive home to Athens was quiet. We didn't attempt to talk. All I could hear was the sound of our car zipping along I-85. Shzzzzzzzzzzzzzzzzzzzzzzzzzzzz.

Chapter 15

Country Roads

I couldn't wait to begin my reeducation. I was strongly encouraged not to use my left-ear hearing aid for six more months, the idea being that it would serve as a crutch and slow my implant learning process. I went about the house as though I were exploring a new world. I opened and closed windows, flipped locks, flushed toilets, and turned on a hair dryer, an electric toothbrush, and a microwave oven. I listened intently, making mental notes. I put my ear close to Cadbury, our big dark-chocolate tomcat, hoping to hear his purring motor. It all sounded like so much white noise, though sometimes there were slight variations. If the phone rang, I might recognize it for what it is, or I might mistake it for Marty turning on the coffee grinder. If she called out to me and was out of my line of vision, I would have to scurry around the house, looking for her. I couldn't tell if she was in the kitchen or in the living room. I couldn't tell if she was upstairs or down. I had no sense of sonic direction.

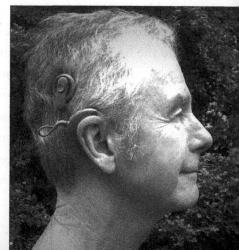

Other days, I felt as though I were wearing a goldfish bowl over my head. A full bowl. I sent out an email update to my sons sarcastically headlined "Welcome to the Undersea World of Noel Cousteau."

I also discovered a dismaying side effect. Once I was off pain-killers and my appetite returned, I discovered I had no sense of taste. Having everything sound like radio static is bad enough. Having everything taste like unadulterated Cream of Wheat was insult on top of injury. I had pondered developing my other senses to make up for the lack of music.

I had been warned, kind of. In her pre-op briefing, Dr. Hoffmann had explained that reaching the cochlea required precision drilling in a crucial, complex area, a junction of all sorts of nerves. Potential damage, while rare, included facial paralysis, blindness, and brain injury. I took the risk. Nobody mentioned the possible loss of taste, however, not that I could recall.

In an email via a secure website through which doctors and patients can communicate privately, Dr. Hoffmann said she was unaware of anyone losing his or her taste after a cochlear operation. She theorized that a nerve had been bruised by the surgery and that my ability to taste food would probably come back.

Probably? I was thinking, *Am I doomed to a life of not being able to distinguish a fried green tomato from a spoonful of peanut butter, except by consistency?*

From the be-thankful-for-small-blessings department, however, there was gravel. I discovered while out for a walk in my neighborhood that I could hear gravel crunch under my feet. It sounded like I remembered crunching gravel sounding. It was a wonderful sound, clean and brisk and real. The nearby gravel, however, was just spillover from a few driveways onto the pavement. We drove out into the boonies outside Athens and found some actual, full-fledged gravel country roads. Every step was a reward.

Technology, meanwhile, was determined to be frustrating. Along with my relearning everyday sounds, Amber Rolfes had insisted that I immediately start using Sound and Way Beyond, a training pro-gram Cochlear Americas developed and includes in its suitcase kits. All I had to do was upload the provided CD-ROM and start doing exercises covering everything from animal and musical-instrument sounds to spoken words. But I couldn't upload the CD without an activation code, and I couldn't get the activation code because Cochlear Americas' server was down. When I went to the company's website, the only means of customer service contact I could find initially was a phone number. But of course, talking on the phone was not an option. This was my first experience of something that I—and no doubt thousands of hearing-impaired people—have come to know as commonplace: companies and offices and services that revolve around the deaf and hearing impaired that don't provide for emails or texts.

Two weeks after my activation, I heard back, via email, from a Cochlear Americas customer rep. The server was up. I uploaded the program and began to do various exercises and take the follow-up tests. There were exercises involving Vowel Recognition, Consonant Recognition, and whole sentences.

In the Consonant Recognition exercise, you're presented with a grid on your computer screen that looks a bit like a Bingo card. There are sixteen alphabetical combinations: aBa, aTa, aLa, aMa, aSHa, aGa, and so on. Various speakers, male and female, some with high, light voices, others with deeper, more resonant timbres, say the various phrases; and you have to click on the phrase on the grid that you believe you heard. You may think "aDa" is easily distinguishable from "aPa." On my first try, I got only eight out of forty correct, and half of those were guesses.

Progress was slow. Very slow. Almost imperceptible. I did Consonant Recognition daily in my office at the Peabodys, shutting my door so my coworkers wouldn't hear the disembodied voices going "ah-Ka," ah-Ba," or the sound of a horse's whinny or a frog's croak. Yes, there was an exercise for learning to identify "everyday" sounds, including animal noises.

Four cartoon drawings at a time would appear on the screen— for instance, a yawning man, a typewriter, a galloping horse, and a fluttering bat. A sound would waft from the computer speaker, and then I would be prompted to click on an image, matching it to the audio clue. When I finished clicking on the twenty-screen test, the Sound and Way Beyond program would automatically give me my score and tell me if I needed to repeat the test or was eligible to move up to a more difficult level. I felt like a kindergartner, a not terribly bright kindergartner, hoping to get a gold star from teacher. Or a kid playing Super Mario Brothers.

There was an exercise for identifying musical sounds, as well. I discovered that I was better at differentiating a mooing cow from a ringing telephone than I was at distinguishing a piano from a flute, but I was better at both than I was with words, the thing I wanted most to hear at that moment.

I was making such poor progress, I had Marty come to my office and take some of the tests. She has, as I have noted, amazing hearing, ears like a barn owl. She found the recorded voices a bit fuzzy, but it was impossible to tell if the problem was the computer's speakers or *my* speakers. I emailed the help desk on the Cochlear Americas website and inquired whether other implantees had complained of the training program audio not being clear. I was told that the program had been thoroughly tested and that complaints were infrequent. Every implantee is different, I was reminded; I just needed to be patient and keep up the training.

To me, perhaps defensively, it sounded as if I were being told that I wasn't trying hard enough. But I was trying hard, I believed. I wanted desperately to be able to engage in something approximating normal conversation.

Was I the problem, or was something not right with my bionic ear gear? I decided it was me, if only because I felt as though I had no other choice. It wasn't as if I could have Dr. Hoffmann jiggle my wiring like it was an extension cord with a short, much less ask Blue Cross Blue Shield to pay for another operation just a month or two after I got my implant.

Chapter 16

Here Comes the Night

W hile my waking hours were a constant quest to match sounds I detected to whichever creature or kitchen appliance was making them, my nights were an auditory void. Bedtime is a strange time for the cochlear-implant dependent, a stretch of peace and paranoia. When you remove the processor from the side of your skull and detach the magnet, you are deaf as a stone. It may not sound like such a bad thing, and in some regards that's true. More than once, Marty griped over morning coffee and raisin bran about our neighbor's "damn dog," barking all night. To which I could honestly say, "What dog?"

Dogs, late-night parties next door, hospital helicopters passing overhead, car alarms—none of it was audible to someone like me when I was unplugged. Then again, neither are tornado sirens, smoke alarms, or the sound of our cats rampaging through the house, knocking over vases and lamps.

Years before I achieved this condition, I wrote a song about insomnia that I called "Maybe It's the Snakes." It's partly a litany of things that you hear or imagine you hear because you can't sleep— or that in fact keep you awake.

"Maybe it's the faucet/dripping down the drain/maybe it's the wailing/in the distance of a train." The title comes from another couplet: "Maybe it's the spiders/maybe it's the snakes/maybe it's that growling sound/the 'frigerator makes."

At the time I wrote it, I kind of dreaded things that go bump or hiss in the night. Now, I longed for them.

Without my artificial ears on, there was nothing there but me and my thoughts. I couldn't wear my left-ear hearing aid to bed. If I rolled over to my left side and pinned it to my pillow, it squealed. The cochlear implant on the other side didn't make that delightful stuck-pig sound, but rolling over and dragging it across the pillow case created a magnified scratching like a club DJ working a turntable. *Psst-tish, sisk-tish, sisk-tish, psst-tish.* Not pleasant, even if you're into hip-hop. And besides, fourteen or fifteen waking hours of having the magnetic cap stuck to your noggin takes a toll. The robotized-sounding voices, the overamplified crash of cabinet doors and cutlery, the roar of white noise at the grocery store or the coffee shop—it gets old. The processor seated behind your outer ear, light though it is, can still leave the skin feeling rubbed raw and sore. The magnet pinches after a while. You need to be detached. You need some quiet time. Or at least you think you do.

Sleeping is fine, the faster it comes and the deeper the better. You may even dream you can hear. But to wake up at three in the morning and not be able to conk out again for an hour or two is like being in a sensory deprivation tank. You're not only deaf, but you are circumstantially blind. Sure, you could turn the lights on, but then your odds of regaining unconsciousness drop off considerably. So you lie there, peering into the darkness, hearing nothing, exploring the crevices between your teeth, tasting the onions from the burger you had for dinner, feeling every itch, and thinking. Thinking, thinking, thinking.

In these stretches of insomnia, my mind free-associates like mad. Worries about money, anxiety about health and aging, doubts about self-worth, confusion about life's purpose and meaning, and

BIG questions roil and mingle with snippets of song lyrics, thoughts about my kids, how they're doing, and why they don't write.

Most of my life, I had used music as a balm and a sedative. Now it was not an option. Marty got me a book about meditation. A daily meditation practitioner herself, she was certain what I needed was a means of quieting an excessively busy brain.

But how can I meditate if I can't hear myself chanting, "Ommm," right? She said I only need to hear it in my mind.

I tried, with only occasional success. Mostly I just let my obsessive-compulsive side take over and make lists. Lists of clothing to take to the cleaners tomorrow. Lists of old movies I could order from Netflix. Lists of places in the world I'd like to visit. Lists of my favorite shortstops of all time. Lists of books I should finally get around to reading (*Paradise Lost, War and Peace, The Da Vinci Code, Fifty Shades of Grey*). Lists of songs with "night" in the title ("Night Moves," "Nights in White Satin," "The Night the Lights Went Out in Georgia," "Goodnight, Irene").

Eventually, I would put myself to sleep.

Chapter 17

Blue Christmas

Christmas was approaching, my first as a guy with only slightly more hearing capacity than a yule log. First and only, I kept telling myself. First and only.

Marty asked me what I wanted for Christmas. "Well, not CDs," I said.

In point of fact, music had been my holiday default for years. I don't use a whole lot of tools that require electricity. I haven't hunted since my Mississippi youth. I don't golf. Fallen arches had long ago put a big crimp in my tennis game. Christmas for me was good chocolate, funny boxer shorts, and new music.

What I wanted most, however, was old music, familiar music. I still have the copy of the Elvis Presley Christmas LP that I found under the tree when I was ten years old. It has a few scratches, but it's still playable, and I wanted to hear it during the season to be jolly, just as I had for decades. No go. I put it on the turntable, but I could barely track the cadence of familiar songs, much less comprehend the melody. I could hear Elvis singing in my head—but what I was missing was not my baby, but my working cochlea.

For years, I had grumbled about the too-early onset of Christmas music, the increasingly inescapable presence not long after Halloween of Johnny Mathis and Bing Crosby crooning yuletide evergreens on the radio, in shops, and in elevators. Now, in my first near-deaf holiday season, I would have been thrilled to hear "Do You Hear What I Hear?" by the Johnny Mann Singers or "The Little Drummer Boy" by the Hollyridge Strings. I would have glowed to the sound of Christmas Muzak.

Elvis's Christmas LP was just part of my long-standing Christmas routine. I have other albums that I have treasured for years, especially *A Nonesuch Christmas,* an amazing sampling of music from the Renaissance and Middle Ages assembled by Nonesuch Records, a label that specialized in offbeat and over-looked classical music; *The New Possibility,* an album of musical meditations on the nativity by guitarist John Fahey; and a Modern Jazz Quartet best-of that included "England's Carol," the combo's celebrated rendition of "God Rest Ye Merry, Gentlemen," and sec-ular MJQ originals like "The Cylinder" and "The Golden Striker" that, in such close association, sounded as holiday-spirited as "Joy to the World."

Starting in early December, I would get up early and do my morning stretches to one of these records. It was my version of advent. I would bathe in the aural ambiance of festivity, calm, and reverence. What I had taken for granted in December 2009 was gone in December 2010. The Nonesuch collection, so harmoni-cally rich, sounded especially dreadful, a sonic mush. I stretched in silence.

We did our best to make up for my silent days and nights with food and sights. We went to a cut-your-own tree farm and sawed down our own evergreen, savoring the clean, piney smell of the saw-dust. We baked cookies and banana bread and made gumbo from an old Mississippi Gulf Coast recipe that takes two days prep and enough crustaceans to feed a seal colony. We went driving all over greater Athens in search of Christmas-decoration extravaganzas, houses outlined from roof peak to hedges in lights, manger scenes, and inflatable snowmen cheek to jowl. We went to a Christmas Eve service at an Episcopal church, a High Mass. The choir sounded like banshees to me, but the clergy were in splendid, full vestment, and the sanctuary was redolent of evergreen boughs and incense. I basked in the service's beatific vibe.

Under our tree on Christmas morning, I found several pairs of really cool socks. Argyle is the new jazz.

Chapter 18

Radiant Beams

In mid-January, Marty and I drove four hours from Athens to Savannah so she could compete in the city's annual American Traditions singing festival, an invitational, juried competition that demands contenders from all across the country to demonstrate their command of multiple genres, from Broadway show tunes to jazz, hymns, and Great American Songbook pop. The late, great tunesmith Johnny Mercer, a Savannah native, is sort of the patron saint of the competition. Marty had participated in 2009, made the semifinals, and come away with enough prize money to cover the cost of our three-day stay. She was determined to try again, not so much for cash possibility, but as an act of defiance, a refusal to let her cancer or my hearing issues dictate our everyday life.

She was so determined, in fact, that she postponed the six weeks of post-op radiation therapy that, if her doctors and her sister Margaret had had their way, would have begun in late December. The radiation specialist had to twist her arm to get her to agree to the treatment at all. Since I was in no condition to be her second set of ears, Margaret had gone with her to the initial consultation. As a nurse, she advocated for the therapy. I did as well, but Marty was insistent.

"I'm only Phase I," she argued, "and my lymph nodes were clear." She relented only after a telephone conversation with another of her sisters, Amy, who was battling a much more serious form of cancer.

"If they missed a single cell," Amy told her, "and if that cell is cancerous, and if it migrates, you'll have to go through all this crap again. Think of this as insurance."

Amy, who lives near Omaha, had gone through gut-wrenching chemotherapy treatments. She's tough stuff and hard to argue with. Plus, she and several other cancer survivors who counseled Marty said that radiation, compared to chemo, was a walk in, well, if not the park, a transitional neighborhood.

Still, it was sing first, get radiated later. We stayed at a friend's condo on Tybee Island and commuted back and forth to the singing competition, the opening rounds of which were held in the sanctuary of a grand old church in Savannah's historic district. Sitting in a front pew, I could hear "sound" as the singers took their turns at the microphone, but without the printed program that told me this barrel-chested guy was performing "Some Enchanted Evening" or that perky woman was singing "On the Atchison, Topeka and the Santa Fe," I hadn't a clue what was coming out of their mouths. I focused on body language.

At least I could imagine what Marty was singing and fill in some blanks, since I knew her repertoire and her animated delivery so well. On the strength of bravura and crowd-pleasing renditions of "Fever" and "Amazing Grace," she once again made it to the semifinals, but also again, no further. She wasn't disappointed. The American Traditions competition is fierce. Many of the contestants are conservatory and university voice professors. She had gotten up on stage and sung her heart out less than three months after undergoing cancer surgery. It was good for her, good for us. Once she was out of the running, we explored more of the old city, took chilly walks on the beach at Tybee, and pretended we were just another off-season vacationing couple, all expenses paid.

Her radiation treatments began almost as soon as we returned to Athens. I wanted to drive her to and from, and several friends offered as well, but here again she was determined to be self-reliant. The Northeast Georgia Cancer Center was only a few miles from our house, and her treatments—one a day, Monday through Friday, for six weeks—proved not to be nauseating. Nor were they exhausting, at least not initially. She maintained a mile-a-day walking schedule at first. By the fifth week, she was sleeping a lot—early to bed, late to rise, with naps in between.

She invited me to her final session, not only to witness the therapy, but to meet staff and fellow patients. People fighting cancer tend to bond, she had told me, women especially. As I shook hands and nodded to acknowledge names I pretended to understand, the camaraderie, fondness even, was unmistakable and touching.

I was invited into the shielded booth to observe. Marty entered the treatment area in a thin, striped gown. A nurse positioned her on a narrow, metal table, then joined me and the radiologist behind the glass. The L-shaped machine that hovered above her looked like the armature of a giant, stainless steel Kitchen Aid mixer. Marty closed her eyes as the room darkened. The table slowly rose, lifting her like a sacrificial offering. If there was whirring, I couldn't hear it, but for the next minute or so, red laser beams coming from several different angles above illuminated the area around her right breast. It was as if she were the besieged heroine of a science-fiction movie and I was an extra. I was more than impressed. I was wowed.

Back in street clothes, in the lobby, she thanked the staff profusely, as did I. Outside, in the car, she told me they and her fellow patients had been incredible, kind, inspiring—and that she hoped she never saw them again unless it was at the grocery store or in line at the multiplex.

Two weeks later, after promising the director she would let her know if she found herself tiring, Marty began rehearsals for *Alice*, a Rose of Athens Theater musical based on *Alice in Wonderland*. She had composed songs and would conduct a vocal orchestra formed by the cast. Life at home was starting to feel almost normal. Almost.

Chapter 19
Dancing in the Dark

O ur love life took a decided downturn after our respective surgeries. We might have been headed for a crystal-anniversary slump under normal circumstances, but Marty's surgery and my hearing problems dealt us a double hit. Physical intimacy was infrequent, and when she did feel like being lovers, it was odd—and I don't mean kinky.

There's an old joke about sex with a condom being like taking a shower wearing a raincoat. Sex without hearing is like going to a concert wearing a space helmet.

Imagining sex without sight isn't difficult. Some people actually prefer to do it under cover of darkness, and most everybody closes his or her eyes some of the time during erotic activity. It can actually be an aphrodisiac to deprive yourself of vision. It can heighten your other senses, increase the feeling of being lost, of abandon.

We were well aware of the drawbacks to my wearing my hearing aid while making love. If anything got too close to that ear—a nose, a hand, a foot, whatever—the hearing aid let out a yelp that's audible, and not just to me. There's nothing like a squealing hearing aid to spoil a mood. Well, other than a squalling baby, perhaps. Ear nibbling, something I have enjoyed since I first experienced it as a spin-the-bottle teen, is a guaranteed squealer. And the same goes for sweet nothings, words of love. Even whispered soft and true, they set off the aid.

Sex without even one good ear is an even greater challenge. Marty told me one of the most lamentable effects of my hearing loss on our love life was its restriction of "pillow talk," before or after. Words and sounds are essential aspects of foreplay, but if I lie next to her on my left side, I lose half my hearing, and the aid yips like a Chihuahua. If I lie next to her on my right side, I lose half my hearing, and the implant processor, though she can't hear it, rubs on the pillow any time I move in the slightest and makes a sound like crinkling paper. And as buzz kills go, responding, "What? Say that again," to a murmured affection or a spontaneous request for more of this or that is on par with hearing aid feedback.

Forget mood music, too. It might as well be cows mooing. Not only does it sound like mush, it also masks hearing what your partner may say. So, no Marvin Gaye, no Anita Baker, no *Out of Africa* soundtrack, no "Season of the Witch."

And that's only for the warm-up. You have to be careful about getting carried away, forgetting yourself, which kind of defeats the purpose. There are maneuvers that can activate the worst possibilities of both hearing devices simultaneously, a squeal in one ear and a scratch like chalk on a blackboard in the other. More than once I've had my implant processor slapped from my ear by my wife's hand and sent flying across the room.

The other option, of course, is to leave all the hardware on the night stand to go "natural" and simply remove sound from your half of the encounter. The upside is that squealing electronics are no longer a worry. The downside is it's much harder to read your partner if you cannot hear words—or sighs or gasps or moans. I never realized how much something as quiet as a whisper, a breath, in my ear mattered, how inspirational it was, until it stopped registering.

I think about "Physical," a hit record singer Olivia Newton-John had years back. "Let me hear your body talk," the pounding, insinuating chorus went. I always assumed the line referred to hearing in the auditory sense, but I've learned as a matter of necessity to hear anatomical articulation in other ways. It's a matter of using other sensors, making yourself alert to changes in temperature, pulse rate, scent, taste, and heartbeat—things I should have been more attuned to all along. So, the big loss ultimately made me more considerate, more engaged, and more receptive.

It also helps, if you don't already, to turn on the lights.

Chapter 20

The Witch Doctor

E ven as Marty was undergoing radiation, I had begun therapy
of my own. The Sound and Way Beyond training program
was driving me nuts and making me angry. In January, I
engaged the services of a professional speech therapist through Athens
Regional Medical Center. The hospital assigned me to Kelly Claas,
a young mother of two who mostly worked with children who were
deaf or had speech disorders. Her suite was strewn with brightly col-
ored blocks and toys. I did insist on a regular, adult-sized chair.

Kelly is not a witch doctor, chapter title notwithstanding. It's
simply that she uses Daniel Ling's "Six-Sound Test," a basic tool of
speech therapy. It includes the sounds "oo," "eee" and "ah."

It reminded me of a popular novelty record of my childhood,
"Witch Doctor," written and performed by David Seville, the guy
who later created Alvin and the Chipmunks. The helium-voiced
chorus is built around those very vowel sounds.

Ling's sound test also covers "mmm," sssss," and "sh." The six
sounds are like keys to the hearing universe. Twice a week, I would
sit in a chair facing Kelly and try my best to train my implant ear
to make sense of spoken sounds and words.

Initially, she would just hide her face behind a little screen on
a wooden stick—like the fans handed out at churches in the South
before air conditioning became common—and patiently present me

with a randomly shuffled mix of "oo," "mmm," "ah, "ssss," "shhh," and "ee." To anyone who hears just fine, it may seem absurd that I had trouble distinguishing "sss" from "shh" or "mmm" from "ah." I certainly thought so, on an intellectual level, but the reality was that it was maddeningly difficult at first.

Even as I worked with Kelly and practiced listening at home—Marty read paragraphs from magazines aloud to me so I couldn't anticipate words—I began to wonder if perhaps there was some virus, some condition still at play in my body. Something that had been missed and gone untreated and that was continuing to have an impact, undermining my progress.

I remembered what my dad had gone through in the year before a specialist in New Orleans found a lemon-sized tumor inside his skull. Doctors in Jackson, Mississippi, had given him a clean bill of health. When his blackouts persisted, he took almost any advice he got, be it AMA approved or folk wisdom. A chiropractor realigned his spine and cracked his neck. He had all four of his wisdom teeth pulled. Informed that a glass of wine every day might improve his blood pressure and ease the headaches and spells, he grudgingly set aside his temperance-union ways. Every evening before supper, he held his nose and dutifully downed half a jelly glass of Mogen David, the only wine he could get in our dry Mississippi county.

Thanks to my MRI, I was pretty confident that I didn't have a tumor. But I embarked on a somewhat similar odyssey, looking for something that might make a difference, that would make the implant kick into gear the way everybody—Amber Rolfes, Dr. Hoffmann, my brother Tim—had expected.

I am not one to give up easily. When I was a boy, a small, scrawny boy—not the strapping five-foot-eight, 140-pound hulk I am now—I loved baseball, which was practically a religion in that Mickey Mantle-Willie Mays era. The summer I was eight, I tried out for a Little League team. I was not picked by any of the coaches. When I was nine, I tried out again, and, again, my parents got no call. At ages ten, eleven, and twelve, same thing. There were few slots to be filled. I kept practicing, played unsupervised sandlot ball whenever I could, played on a Little League "farm" team on which my teammates, great guys, included a boy who'd had polio when he was younger and a kid who'd shot his right eye out with a BB gun. When I tried out for a Babe Ruth League team when I was thirteen, a coach who lived in my neighborhood picked me. I was ecstatic. And I sat the bench, never played a single inning, until the final game of the season, when my team had the pennant clinched. When I was sent in to pinch-hit late in the game with two men on base, the opposing pitcher, a hefty fifteen-year-old, mocked me by motioning for his outfielders to come in close. I hit his third pitch over the center fielder's head for a ground-rule double and strolled into second base.

The following season I was the starting shortstop. The season after that, I made the all-star team. I am not one to give up easily.

I was game to try anything that might boost my ability to hear. I had acupuncture, lying in a chaise longue in a quiet room with dozens of tiny needles stuck in my ear lobes and neck. I became a client of an alternative, holistic clinic, getting massages and practicing deep breathing. They encouraged me to go gluten-free. Perhaps it was pasta and French bread that were poisoning my ears. I cut out both, and we began baking our own breads with rice and soy flours. I lost almost ten pounds in a month, but my hearing got no better. Like my mysteriously ill father before me, I tried a chiropractor. My tight neck got better. My ears did not. One thing I didn't do that my dad did was drink wine. I'm not a teetotaler like he was, but booze of any kind tended to dull the hearing in my still-natural left ear. So did eating hot dogs or salami, anything high in salt and nitrates. I got healthier, albeit inadvertently, just not much better at understanding words.

More and more I wondered: Is the problem not me at all? Is it the equipment?

***

Meanwhile, I sensed that I was losing my identity.

"How's your hearing?"

The question was becoming a joke. A bad joke. If I bumped into somebody I knew at the grocery store, encountered neighbors on a stroll around the horseshoe cul-de-sac where we live, or joined a party, "How's your hearing?" was almost always the first thing I would be asked. And quite often, the last.

Serious hearing loss redefines you. It overshadows everything else about you that makes you "you." I still read newspapers and all sorts of magazines, still had opinions, still went canoeing and bird-watching, and still checked out new restaurants in town. But hardly anybody seemed to care anymore.

I was now Hearing-Impaired Guy. I was Mos Deaf. People would inquire how I/it was doing honestly, earnestly, with perfectly good intentions. And I would tell them. At first, I tended to tell them at length, but I soon learned to condense my updates. This was partially because I would notice that Marty, wearing a "not again" expression, was distancing herself from me and whomever I was talking to, and partially because I could "hear" myself falling into recitation of overused lines, like an author on a book tour who had done one too many interviews on local radio stations.

But even after I started to keep my answers shorter, "How's your hearing?" was at once a conversation starter and stopper. Maybe some people were made uncomfortable by my disability. Maybe, after the courtesy of asking, they couldn't help pulling away when they realized how tricky it would be to have a true give-and-take. Maybe I was just becoming a bore.

I hated it. Deafness was making me invisible.

Chapter 21
Hello, It's Me

Marty and I were grocery shopping at the neighborhood supermarket when a man about my age approached us in the pasta aisle. He mouthed something that I could not understand. Marty translated. He had noticed my implant. He turned his head and pointed. He had one, too.

He and Marty carried on a conversation while I watched. He pulled a business card from his wallet and gave it to her, nodding toward me. He was a University of Georgia professor. In an email exchange the next day, he told me about his hearing loss and implantation. I asked how he fared in his classes. He said he sometimes had trouble understanding students speaking from the back rows, but otherwise he did just fine. He told me to have patience, better word comprehension would come.

My patience was being sorely tested. It was six months after my activation, and the most positive development I could point to was that my sense of taste had returned. I had homemade pesto and sweet potato pie to help me stay sane. Without my left-ear hearing aid for support, I could follow only the simplest conversation—and even then, only in a quiet, acoustically perfect room. Amber Reith had brought in a Cochlear Americas field representative to assist her in a mapping session. Still, the predicted clarity did not arrive.

I had met another implantee while accompanying Marty on a breast-cancer charity walk. His wife was a survivor, too. Dr. Steenerson had done the man's implant. Marty told them about the struggle I was having. He could hear. He encouraged me to make an appointment with the cochlear audiologist on Dr. Steenerson's staff, Cindy Gary. He said she was the best and most experienced in the state, not to mention a sweetheart of a human being.

With Amber Rolfes' blessing, I made an appointment with Cindy. We started the mapping process over again from scratch. One of the first things she noticed was that five electrodes, all on the outermost end of the array, were getting weak responses or none at all when she tested them. One explanation, she said, would be that they hadn't made it into my cochlea. Marty told her about Dr. Hoffman's having met with "resistance" when inserting the array.

Great, I thought. I'd done some reading. A healthy human has some 15,000 hair cells, about 20 percent of which—3,500—directly transfer information to the brain. A perfectly working implant, with all of its twenty-two electrodes functioning, can approximate only a tiny fraction of that. And here I was with almost a fourth of *my* electrodes cooling their heels on the patio outside my cochlea.

Cindy assured us that while this situation was not ideal, she could adjust the mapping to accommodate the missing electrodes. After an exhausting session of more than two hours, I settled on a new map. Cindy tested me by speaking with her mouth hidden from me behind one of those church-fan cardboard squares. I was able to understand most of what she said with no lip-reading assistance. Marty and I headed for the parking lot encouraged.

Yet, by the time we got onto the freeway, I was already having difficulty understanding Marty. We couldn't write it off to road noise, either. At home, in a quiet room, I simply couldn't understand words as well as I had at the ear clinic two hours earlier. What was supposed to happen was that I would comprehend more and more as I acclimated to a new map. Instead, I experienced decline.

And this soon became identifiable as a pattern. It was as though my implant were an old piano that lost its pitch soon after the tuner packed up his tools and left: Cindy would remap me. We'd converse freely in her office. I would go home, and the clarity would fade.

Marty and I wondered whether something was still wrong with me systemically, something as yet undetected that was rendering the implant less effective, or whether the implant itself might be a problem.

Outside Cindy's office on a subsequent visit, we bumped into a middle-aged woman who had the next appointment. I could barely understand her, but she and Marty carried on a lively conversation for two or three minutes. In the elevator, Marty leaned in to my left ear and told me the woman had not one but two implants and conversed so naturally it was impossible to tell there was anything wrong with her ears. I was encouraged. Also envious.

Meanwhile, my efforts to find implantees online with whom I could compare notes had turned up Blue McConnell, a musician in North Carolina. Blue said it had taken her time and practice, but she was back performing again. *With other musicians.* My implant-modulated pitch was so poor, I couldn't sing "Twinkle, Twinkle, Little Star" with Marty without sounding like a cat undergoing torture.

By April 2011, we had decided it was time to get serious about pressing for a reevaluation. Testing for allergies had turned up nothing. Neither had tests for viruses. Maybe I had a faulty implant. Or maybe there was a problem with the surgery. Something wasn't right, and I knew in my heart that it wasn't a matter of me not trying hard enough.

I emailed Dr. Hoffmann by way of NextMD, a password-protected portal through which doctors and patients can communicate with privacy. I wrote:

I continue to struggle with understanding words with my implant. I'm using the Sound and Way Beyond program and work with a speech therapist two times each week, but I still feel like I'm listening to a radio not quite tuned to the station I want to hear or as though I am trying to eavesdrop through a closed door or a wall.

About ten days ago, I tried a different cochlear audiologist (Cindy Gary). We spent four hours on mapping, but the improvement, so far, has been slight. She told me that she got no response from the first four electrodes, suggesting that they are not in the cochlea but, rather, the middle ear. She said only a CT scan would confirm that, however.

If that's in fact the case, would it have any bearing on my difficulty understanding words?

Dr. Hoffmann authorized the CT scan. An MRI would have been better, but that was out of the question now that I had metal in my skull. The first try, on May 11, was at St. Mary's Hospital in Athens, which Blue Cross Blue Shield insisted I use because it was in my HMO plan. The technician had never actually seen an implant before. She went sort of Gomer Pyle over it. *Gaaaaaw-lay.* She summoned colleagues over to show them. I felt like a sideshow attraction, a two-headed calf.

She scanned my head from several different angles. She said the film would be sent to Dr. Hoffmann within a day or two. I let her know via NextMD email, and she replied immediately that she would let me know as soon as she had reviewed the film.

That was that, I figured. Mission accomplished. I directed my attention to preparations for the Peabody Awards ceremony in New York on May 23—the seventieth in the program's history and my first as a "bionic" PR man. It was easier than the previous year's stint in Manhattan, when I was still attempting to prop up my natural ears with daily steroids. At planning sessions with the hotel, it was still as if I were watching TV with the mute button on—mouths moving in animated silence across the table from me. But one-on-one and up close, I could understand at least some of what my colleagues said to me.

We barely had time to get settled back in Athens before it was time to head for Marty's annual family reunion in Nebraska.

She's one of fourteen kids, so the much-generational assemblage is only slightly smaller and less noisy than the Peabody soiree. And it seemed as though every in-law, niece, and cousin wanted to see and ask about this thing on the side of my head and inquire as to my welfare. Only upon our return to Athens did I remember I had heard nothing regarding my CT scan.

On June 23, I emailed Dr. Hoffmann. On July 1, she replied, reporting via NextMD that the scan had showed that the implant was "clearly" in the cochlea.

"The radiology report noted that it is about 8–9 mm past the cochleostomy," she said. "There is no way to tell about the position of any individual electrodes, as there is not enough detail on the film and the electrodes are microscopic. It appears that most of the implant is in place. I hope this is helpful."

Helpful, sort of. Satisfying, not really. But I decided to tough it out. We had a long-scheduled visit to Florida coming up. We were going to see some of my old *Orlando Sentinel* colleagues and go bird-watching on Sanibel Island off the Gulf Coast near Ft. Myers. In the quiet of my former editor's den in Orlando, I had the most intelligible conversation I'd had in months. At a dinner party at another old friend's home, I nodded and pretended to understand even as the lively dinner chatter pounded my ears so hard they rang for hours afterward. It was that unpredictable from day to day.

On Sanibel, it didn't matter nearly so much. The island is famously slow-paced and quiet even in the high season, and this was the low. The Sanibel speed limits are a crawl. Most residents and visitors bicycle. There are "Turtle Crossing" signs along the roads, and you are expected to heed them. The beaches are beautiful and shell-strewn, the Gulf waters clear and warm, and the waterfowl varied and plentiful. We saw herons, ibis, and roseate spoonbills. It was a smorgasbord for my other senses. Even my limited ears could pick up the sound of the birds. I wanted to plant a flag and build myself a nest.

Chapter 22

Revise and Consent

In mid-September, a friend alerted me to an article in the *Wall Street Journal.* Cochlear Ltd., Cochlear Americas' Australian parent company, was recalling almost forty million dollars' worth of Nucleus 5s—not the thousands, like mine, that were already in people's heads all over the world, but those 5s remaining in inventories—in the wake of an unexplained increase in failures. The failure rate was less than 1 percent, but Cochlear Ltd. was being proactive. The company would revert to marketing its previous state-of-the-art model, the Nucleus Freedom and in fact offer Freedoms free to people who needed to have a 5 replaced.

Cochlear Ltd.'s stock price dropped. My hopes skyrocketed. There was apparently no danger. My Nucleus 5 wasn't going to explode in my head or catch on fire, but maybe it was the source of my difficulties.

It turned out to be a false alarm where I was concerned. The malfunction didn't entail poor performance. The flawed 5s were just quitting on people. Mine had never stopped working. It just didn't work as well as I wanted.

During this stretch, I was flitting between mapping sessions with Cindy Gary at Dr. Steenerson's office and Piedmont's Amber Rolfes. For the former, I had to pay out of pocket. Amber was covered by insurance. For a session with her in September, Amber had

Cochlear Americas's southeastern rep sit in. I complained during the mapping that I *felt* a painful throbbing sensation when some of the electrodes were triggered even though I couldn't hear any beeping. They found that the first seven electrodes in the array of twenty-two were not getting an auditory response. The Cochlear rep wondered if the fluctuations of my hearing might be the result of some systemic problem. I asked Amber to send Dr. Hoffmann a memo about all this rather than risk me misrepresenting the facts.

Dr. Hoffmann soon thereafter emailed me that after having consulted with the Cochlear Americas rep, she thought it would be a good idea to have the company's chief medical officer look at my scan.

On December 8, one of Hoffmann's assistants mailed to say that Cochlear's Dr. Peter Weber had called her a few days earlier. She said that both he and a neuroradiologist on staff had reviewed my scan.

"Although the positioning looks adequate," she reported, "he cannot say if the electrode had folded over slightly or could have been migrating out of the cochlea. He recommended a plain-film X-ray for further evaluation."

I had the X-ray done, again using St. Mary's Hospital in Athens, as instructed by Blue Cross Blue Shield. On the 21st, I got an email from Hoffmann's office. The assistant said that the report indicated that a mastoid scan had been done, but the film included was a chest X-ray.

"Do you remember what they X-rayed at your appointment"? she asked.

I emailed back that unless the technician had very bad aim, it was my head that had been X-rayed—from a variety of angles. She suggested I call St. Mary's and ask them what happened.

I couldn't call, of course, so I had to go to the hospital's billing department, take a number, and wait to see a customer service rep. They eventually found the X-rays of my head and sent them to Hoffmann's office. I was happy to learn somebody's lungs were fine.

Shortly after New Year's, Hoffmann emailed to say that she had gotten a call from Cochlear Americas's Weber. She said he'd had a chance to review the X-ray and noted that it was overexposed and not particularly useful.

"He reports that he cannot see the tip of the electrode," she said. "I did report to him that we had obtained a film at Piedmont Hospital at the time of surgery, and we can compare any other films to that one done initially. It would be helpful to know if the electrode is still in an adequate position. We can repeat the film at Piedmont if you would like to come to Atlanta. Dr. Weber also said that we may consider replacing the implant with revision surgery."

Revision surgery? A do-over? Marty and I each did a double take. Are they finally going to acknowledge that this isn't just a matter of me not trying hard enough to understand simple speech?

Hoffmann's office arranged for me to have yet another X-ray at a facility in Atlanta that Piedmont ENT often used.

I dutifully drove the sixty-five miles to Atlanta and had the new X-ray done. On February 27, I emailed Hoffmann: "If you haven't heard back from Dr. Weber, please press him to weigh in on my X-ray," I wrote. "Someone needs to make my case a priority. I am having trouble functioning at work, and I am having an increasingly difficult time understanding my wife, whose voice is the easiest for me. I need information so I can act on this problem, the sooner the better."

On March 1, she replied:

I was able to talk with Dr. Weber. He feels that the tip of the implant may be folded over. It is unclear if that would explain the fluctuation in your hearing. He recommends removing the implant and replacing it with revision surgery. Because they have pulled your current implant from the market, it would mean replacing it with the Nucleus Freedom, which has a very good track record.

Although I have experience with the initial cochlear implant surgery, I have not had to revise many. I am happy to discuss and perform the revision surgery if you would like, but I also understand if you would like to discuss this with another surgeon. Here are the otologists who perform cochlear implants in the Atlanta area.

I had to sit for a minute to take this news in. Weber had flat out recommended a revision.

I was game. Marty was gamer. But, as we soon learned, this was no simple matter. It wasn't as though I could zip over to Hoffmann's office—or Steenerson's—and have the thing in my head popped out and replaced like a battery for my wristwatch. And getting Blue Cross Blue Shield of Georgia to approve another big-ticket surgery would likely be more complicated than getting the company to okay a second visit to my dermatologist to check on a worrisome mole.

Just *how* complicated, we were about to find out.

Dr. Hoffmann in effect ruled herself out. She didn't say outright that she wouldn't attempt the revision, but her less-than-whole-hearted enthusiasm, along with the fact that she had provided me with a list of alternative surgeons, made our decision easy.

I wanted Dr. Steenerson. He's the most revered cochlear surgeon in Atlanta and probably the whole Southeast, and I couldn't help feeling that if he had been allowed to do the original implant, I might not be in the fix I was in. But Blue Cross Blue Shield had said no in 2010, and there was no guarantee the company would see the revision surgery any differently—if it was approved at all.

Armed with letters from Cochlear Americas's medical officer, Hoffmann, and my primary care physician, Dr. Eric Robach, that attested to the reality and extent of my disability, Blue Cross did, after numerous phone calls from Marty and faxes from me, okay the redo. Just not Steenerson.

Blue Cross's rep said there were other otology specialists presumably capable of doing an implantation who were in my HMO plan. The company would pay for Steenerson to do it only if all the other cochlear specialists in my coverage area—basically, all of Georgia—said they couldn't do it or didn't care to try.

I felt like Captain Ahab trying to finish off Moby Dick. It crossed my mind that I should just give in and let the whale take me under. But Marty, bless her, applied yet another boot to my posterior.

"If they think they can just wear us down and we'll go away, they are sadly mistaken," she said.

I went beyond the list Dr. Hoffmann had provided. I went to Blue Cross's website and wrote down the name, address, and phone number of every otologist and ENT in the state that was in my HMO plan. We started working our way through the list. If he or she had listed an email address or fax number, I made the overture. If there was only a phone number—and this, weirdly enough given that these are doctors who deal with the hearing impaired daily, was often the case—Marty would call.

It was time-consuming but relatively easy. Most of the ear specialists on the list didn't do cochlear implants at all, and those who did expressed no interest in attempting to redo another surgeon's work. One in-plan doctor indicated agreed to take a look at me and my records: Dr. Morton Pendorff.

We were jazzed. I mean, he was veteran surgeon at a well-regarded clinic with an impressive website. And he was not only on Hoffmann's list, he was on the list Steenerson's office had given me back in 2010 when I chose Hoffmann.

Marty phoned the practice to make an appointment. The earliest date we could get was six weeks later. Once again we're going, "Geez, is this going to drag on forever?"

Answer: yes.

To make sure we could find our way to an early morning appointment, we drove to the clinic on the outskirts of Atlanta to scope out the building and the parking situation. We also picked out a motel close by and made a reservation so we would not have to leave at four or five in the morning to make sure we didn't get held up in the metro Atlanta traffic and end up missing the early morning appointment. I also signed and faxed to the office a form granting them permission to acquire my records from Hoffmann, Steenerson, and any other doctor I had seen since March 2010.

We drove to our chosen motel the afternoon before the appointment, had a nice dinner at a little Thai restaurant nearby, got to bed at a decent hour, and headed for the clinic the next morning. Even early in the day, the waiting room was packed. Compared to the gracious staff at Piedmont ENT, the women behind the reception desk at Pendorff's office were about as pleasant as the clerks at a Long Island Department of Transportation office. More than an hour passed before my name was called.

We waited some more in an examination room. While a nurse was taking my pulse and blood pressure, an assistant came in looking irritated and asked if she could have my records. Interpreting for me, Marty said, "What do you mean 'Where are his records?'? We faxed you the form you sent us authorizing you to request them." The assistant said no, we were supposed to bring them with us. Marty said, "No, you were authorized to request them." The assistant argued that we had misunderstood. Marty said, "Well, if that's the case, why did you have us sign and send back that form?"

Before this disagreement turned uglier, the doctor arrived. He made Steenerson seem as convivial as Mr. Rogers. He was gruff and impatient, and when he was told I didn't have my records with me, he was visibly annoyed. He was also under the mistaken impression that I only wanted my implant extracted. No, Marty told him, Cochlear Americas recommended that my implant be *replaced*. He did not seem embarrassed that he didn't understand why I had come to see him, despite the fact that Marty had made it very clear when she made the appointment. He agreed to look at my ear and hear a synopsis of my history anyway, but first he sent me off to one of his audiologists for a hearing test while he mulled it over. He didn't just mull, however. He called Hoffmann for a quick briefing. And Marty, whose hearing is almost as sharp as mine is dull, overheard him out in the hallway telling a nurse that he didn't expect to have any more success than Hoffmann did with getting the array all the way into my cochlea.

The audiologist looked as though she were only a few years out of high school. When she found out that I'd been getting mapped by both Amber Rolfes at Piedmont and Cindy Gary at Steenerson's clinic, she went into lecture mode. She told us that if Dr. Pendorff agreed to tackle my revision, there would be none of this "hopping around." She said she and she alone would do my mapping.

When Marty translated this for me, I just nodded. But I knew what she was thinking and I agreed: No way would I "go steady" with this upstart if her mapping didn't work for me. I would do what I needed to do.

It turned out, however, that she was irrelevant. Dr. Pendorff said that he would see me again if I wanted to come back—and this time with my records—but that his initial take on my problem, given what I and Hoffmann had told him, was that the chances of improvement were slim.

We decided to make another appointment. He was, after all, my last in-plan possibility. Marty discovered that we couldn't get a follow-up until September 26, and the clerk acted as if she were doing us a favor to get us in that soon.

Both of us were livid. On the drive back to Athens, we decided that we were going to see Dr. Steenerson and see what he said. If we had to pay the bill ourselves, maybe we would, even if we have to mortgage the house. We were sick of the monkey business, the seemingly endless bureaucratic crap.

Chapter 23
CapTales

With hearing loss so pervasive now, it's hardly surprising that there are all sorts of gadgets on the market to help us cope with everyday life. As the uncertainty of my recovery sank in, I ordered a catalog, thick as a small-town phone book, from which you can send away for an amazing array of gizmos, including an alarm clock that would shake your bed instead of buzzing and signs for your home street that declare, "Caution: Deaf Person."

I mail-ordered a doorbell that would set off a flashing light like a police cruiser's inside the house. I could ignore phone calls while Marty was out, knowing the answering machine would catch them, but it seemed like a good idea for me to know when someone was at the front door. It might be a neighbor wanting to tell me she'd seen a coyote looking for a snack cat.

I installed the push button outside our front door and plugged the device into an electrical outlet in the kitchen. It produced a high-pitched noise that never failed to startle Marty and freak out the cats, as well as a blinding blinking that always made me feel as though we were about to have a close encounter of the third kind.

I also decided to try the captioning telephones I'd read about. I ordered a CapTel® for home use in April 2011 and a second for my office not long thereafter. The CapTel is a telephone that comes equipped with a display screen. Calls are routed through a service that uses a combination of voice-recognition software and human transcribers to present a deaf person with a running translation of what the other party on the line is saying. In some states, including Georgia, there are government programs in place to subsidize the purchase of a CapTel, lowering the cost to less than one hundred dollars. And the service itself is free.

Like close-captioned TV, however, the captioning phone is a great boon that works better in theory than practice. I quickly discovered it's at its best when the person you are conversing with has the diction of a trained Shakespearean actor, sticks to simple information, and keeps sentences short. If Maggie Smith or Hugh Bonneville phoned me, we'd likely have a jolly good chat, at least at the outset. Even people who possess the needed qualities and start off with the best intentions often drift unconsciously into normal conversational patterns. And it's most unfortunate for southerners that a drawl tends to throw off the machine, as well.

After my mother passed away in 2003, I started phoning my elderly Aunt Nell, my second mom, every evening for a short chat. She and my widowed mom had been roommates for many years, and now she was by herself in a fairly large old house. What began out of concern for her grieving settled into ritual. I would tell her what Marty and our kids were up to, and she would tell me the latest news and gossip in Laurel. We had to take a hiatus after my hearing crashed—I sent her a lot of cards and letters instead—but we resumed the ritual when I got my captioning phone. She likes to hear my voice, and it comes through loud and clear to her. The CapTel works as well as a regular phone in that regard.

On my end on the line, it's a different story. Not only does she have a classic Southern accent, but she also has a tendency to stream-of-consciousness speech. She rivals William Faulkner for elongated sentences, and she changes topics on a dime. She can utterly confound CapTel. Even when she makes a concerted effort to talk slow, the software—or the transcriber—often mistranslates her words hilariously.

"We had the most delicious ice cream cones" appears on my little screen as "the most siliceous ice cream coats."

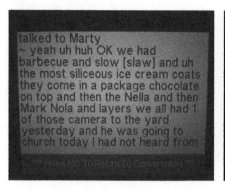
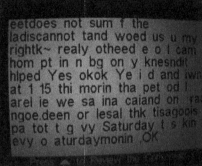

Bragging about a visit from her great-grand niece, she said, "I tell you she does not miss a trick." But the CapTel garbles it into "miss eight track sheep."

It's a never-ending source of amusement, especially when the CapTel misprints this unstintingly proper Methodist lady's words as the bluest profanity, and a frequent source of vexation.

I do better with my sons and my brother, all of whom have deep, resonant voices and enunciate well, but CapTel chatting is still most effective when the person on the other end of the line keeps it unnaturally slow and simple. The longer I had a CapTel, the less I used it for anything other than my aunt and the most necessary calls, like checking my credit card balances. CapTel loves the computer-generated voice of VISA.

Chapter 24

I Say a Little Prayer

In 1973, when I was the *Orlando Sentinel*'s newly commissioned TV-radio columnist, the local public-TV outlet was one of a handful of stations in the national PBS system to broadcast a production of Bruce Jay Friedman's off-Broadway play *Steambath*. The bathhouse was a stand-in for purgatory. A motley assortment of men and women clothed only in white towels killed time trading life stories and philosophies. Meanwhile, a testy Puerto Rican janitor used a bank of TV monitors to randomly keep watch over various people on Earth and arbitrarily afflict them with cancer or arrange fatal, head-on freeway collisions. He ordered acne for Debbie Reynolds.

It was satire, of course, a rueful joke. I don't know if Friedman believed in any kind of God, but it was clear he didn't believe the heartache, hard luck, and pain we all encounter during our limited time on Earth is ordained or orchestrated by a vengeful or contrary creator.

I mention *Steambath* because I have never thought of my hearing loss as divine recompense for something I did wrong or didn't do right. Well, maybe momentarily a few times. It's hard not to wonder. But as a long-haul rationale, no. It is what it is, so deal with it.

Religiously speaking, I've spent most of my adult life as what an old college buddy called a "Seventh Day Adventurer." I was raised Methodist and still go back to it from time to time. John Wesley is one of my namesakes. But I have dabbled over time in everything from Judaism to Buddhism. I was occasionally attending services at the Unitarian Universalist Fellowship of Athens at the time of my hearing loss. My wife and I are members there now.

I haven't prayed to be delivered from this disability, and I haven't asked friends or family to do so on my behalf. If they want to on their own, wonderful. I appreciate the love and good and positive energy it represents. But I don't count on it to cure my problem, a pretty niggling ailment, actually, given all the possibilities. It's not that I don't "believe" in the practice, just that I don't think my mind is now or ever will be big enough or acute enough to grasp whatever Big Picture there might be.

I wrote a song that addresses this idea some years ago. Marty and I were driving up the Natchez Trace, a quiet Mississippi highway that follows an ancient Native American path from Vicksburg up through Jackson to Nashville. Somewhere around Tupelo, where we hoped to see Elvis's birthplace and possibly the phantom king himself, I had a flash of inspiration while listening to a gospel radio station. Marty was napping on the passenger side when I pulled off the Trace, found a ballpoint and an empty envelope in the glove compartment, and jotted down the lyrics buzzing around in my head. It took no more than ten minutes. It's about what we pray for and how. I eventually called it "These Things."

> *Give us this day our daily bread*
> *Stop the roof from leaking over our heads*
> *And don't let us be too easily led*
> *These things we ask of you*
>
> *Watch over our souls while we're asleep*
> *Keep the price of tomatoes from climbing too steep*
> *Make the rest of our years always be leap*
> *These things we ask of you*

These things we ask of you, dear Lord
These things we ask of you
We'll get by somehow if you don't come through
But these things we ask of you

Bow heads at the table, kneel by our beds
We think with our hearts, we thank with our heads
But you're in the black, Lord, and we're in the red
These things we ask of you

These things we ask of you, dear Lord
These things we ask of you
We'll get by somehow if you don't come through
But these things we ask of you

We fall on our faces, we fall on our knees
We know, dear Lord, you do as you please
Help us to tell the woods from the trees
These things we ask of you

These things we ask of you, dear Lord
These things we ask of you
We'll get by somehow, we always do
But these things we ask of you

I haven't got a clue whether my hearing loss or any other adversity I've ever faced is "personal" or if it's part of some larger plan like, oh, prompting me to write a book. When I pray—and I do—it's never for things, just for patience and perspective.

Chapter 25
Realm of the Senses

I hit upon a new coping strategy: sensorial diversity.

I was a big fan of Marvel comics when I was a teenager, and none of Stan Lee's imperfect superheroes intrigued me more than Daredevil, a blind crime fighter who had developed his other senses, not to mention his reflexes, to prodigious heights to compensate for his inability to see. As I came to realize that I might never regain anything approaching full hearing and that what I did regain might well be erratic and spotty, I started thinking about Daredevil and his triumph of will.

I was a little old for gymnastics and martial arts training. I wasn't even playing basketball anymore because of fallen arches. Still, I stepped up my exercise regimen at the Y, betting that with patience, consistency, and a lack of vanity when it came to deciding how much weight to lift, I could get myself back into shape for more adventurous hiking, perhaps even running. It would be good to feel the air rushing past my face and arms again.

The goal wasn't to develop super senses, but to indulge those that were not impaired. If new music sounded like ugly sonic mush, I could indeed stop and smell the roses. And the coffee. And the baking bread. I could crush a few leaves of rosemary or basil between my thumb and forefinger and inhale the fragrance, an olfactory wake-up call. I could get high on the aroma of garlic and onions slowly sautéed in olive oil. I could breathe the scent of Marty's hair in the night.

If I yearned for freewheeling conversation, I could treat myself to a premium chocolate bar, order the orgasmic escargot at Athens's one-and-only French bistro, or eat a Vietnamese or Greek dish I had never tried before. I could detour off the Interstate and onto a Georgia back road that would lead me to a roadside stand selling heirloom peaches, exquisitely flavorful beneath their thick, old-fashioned fuzz. I could have a slab of vine-ripened tomato with sea salt and a dash of mayo. I could make my mom's gumbo.

If I couldn't make a phone call, I could feel the shock and thrill of a sudden dive into a cool swimming pool. Like the B52s sang, I could "dance in the garden in torn sheets in the rain." I could invest in Egyptian cotton sheets with a sinfully high thread count. I could start treating massage as a necessity, not a luxury. I could take a tip from my wife, an apparel hedonist, and buy some clothes strictly for the feel of them.

If I felt deprived of aural stimulation, I could use my two reasonably good eyes to see more than I had been seeing. Just as our brains learn to screen out sounds that aren't necessary, so it is with our vision.

What's the Bible verse? There is none so blind as he who will not see? It's true. We can become so narrowly or tightly focused that the wider world becomes a blur. One of the reasons nature documentaries can be so compelling is that the filmmakers focus for us. They share their observational powers. They direct our eyes. But we are capable of doing this for ourselves, albeit not exotically. Our own backyards are teeming with natural wonder if we stop, get still, and really, truly look. There are remarkably intricate mushrooms and lichens near my house that I barely noticed before I adopted the Daredevil approach. There are little green lizards that flash pink throat pouches and shiny, black-and-blue skinks that are too gorgeous for such an inelegant name. And now that I have trained my eye to pay more attention, I not only see vastly more birds—cardinals, flickers, cedar waxwings, purple buntings—flitting around the trees off my back deck, but hawks on power lines or in dead trees along the highway and egrets fishing in roadside ditches and ponds. How many years did I look right past them? Now they are the music I drive to.

Museums and art galleries likewise have come into sharper focus. I've always loved museums. The Lauren Rogers Museum in my Mississippi hometown was a great source of childhood pleasure and learning for me, an eclectic treasure trove of Choctaw basketry, European oil paintings, and twentieth-century folk art. With the onset of my hearing loss, I made it a resolution to seek out and closely observe visual art, from Athens street-corner mascot sculptures—bulldogs done up by artists as everything from bankers to Carmen Miranda—to Harold Rittenberry's wrought-iron folk art to a Salvador Dalí exhibit at Atlanta's High Museum.

On a visual-stimulation excursion to the Georgia Museum of Art, an especially magnetic destination because it's on the edge of the University campus and free of charge except for a suggested three-dollar donation, I was delighted to discover a competition in progress. The museum houses a selection of Renaissance paintings donated by the Kress Foundation, named for the five-and-ten-cent store magnate, a prodigious collector. For purposes of the project, everyone who viewed the paintings in the Kress gallery was encouraged to create new art—a painting, a sculpture, a video, a story, a song, a photograph—in response to one or more of the pieces.

I settled on a painting, a Crucifixion tableau by Paolo Schiavo, a fourteenth-century Florentine painter, and returned a few days later to sit and quietly observe it. I turned off my battery-powered ears. I ended up composing a prose poem. What surprised me was not how much there was to see, but how much, when I concentrated and imagined, that there was to hear.

I submitted it under the title "Listening to Art":

I came to you because I'd gone deaf
Not that I expected any healing, mind you
I don't believe in miracles
Not big ones anyway
I didn't even know you were present
In these gleaming pine corridors
Hobnobbing with saints who say they knew you
No, I came because I made myself a New Year's resolution:
"Celebrate the senses you have left, son. Indulge.
Nuzzle that glorious velvet, trace an old hickory's furrowed bough.
Savor that wild strawberry, that kiss of mint.
Smell the roses and the coffee, of course. And the sour mash ferment
Of sweet gum leaves and carrot shavings making compost cider.
Watch the sunrise blossom, the waxwings dining by the open window.
Look at art. Yes! And really look this time."
And so it was that I came to this ivory hall, seeking a feast for my eyes
Not you, just a three-buck all-you-can-eat.
But there you were, in that Florentine's ferocious miniature,
A king embracing eternity between thieves, dying for their sins, our sins
Dying for your decency, for your inability to betray your loving heart.
What a sensory magnificence.
Schiavo's palette burned my eyes, his reds dark like your last cup of wine, like blood I have given
I could feel the rough timber beneath your pale limbs
I inhaled sorrow, tasted triumph.
And I could hear
The Romans grousing, debating your paternity
The sobs that had welled inside your mother for 30 years
Magdalene's words of comfort
There, there. Sssssssh.

Calvary was alive, aural, a cacophony.
I could hear it.
For a moment I could hear.

Scrutinizing and savoring art is a sensory experience, and so, I now understand, is writing, which for so many years was for me a means to an end. But so, too, are a near infinite number of things we do, from building a birdhouse to bricking a patio, from planting bulbs and seeds to inhaling the fragrance of simmering spaghetti sauce. It's all in how you approach these "routine" experiences. Expanding their variety and making them fresh and meaningful to yourself, that's the way you do it, that's how you cope.

Chapter 26
Fight Club

In late July, I went to see Dr. Steenerson. After examining my implanted ear, he agreed to attempt the revision surgery. "Attempt" was the operative word. He expected the operation to be tricky. To avoid the resistance that Dr. Hoffmann had reported encountering, he said he might have to do a sort of "back-door" approach and a "split" electrode array in order to maximize placement. He told me, through Marty, about a woman he had helped who had difficult bone structure. He was so intrigued and perplexed by my predicament that he said he would do the operation for a lower, out-of-pocket fee if BCBS declined to cover it.

We set a November 26 date for my pre-op, with the surgery to take place on December 6.

Marty called Dr. Pendorff's office at Emory and canceled my follow-up appointment.

Meanwhile, Blue Cross denied my request for the revision, stating in a letter that it wasn't "medically necessary."

Marty and I were ready to take advantage of Georgia's liberal gun purchase laws. Not medically necessary? Were they freaking kidding? I couldn't even talk to them on the phone, and they were acting as though I wanted them to cover getting a tattoo removed.

Via NextMD, I emailed Dr. Hoffmann. I told her that I was appealing my case to Blue Cross and that I would appreciate her writing a letter of support, endorsing my need and Dr. Weber's recommendation.

"I'm not sure what medically necessary means, but the revision is functionally essential for me," I said. "My hearing range with the implant is about two feet, and even that close, words are fuzzy and indistinct. I'm useless at meetings and in class. My wife has to pass me notes at dinner. We're learning to sign."

Hoffmann had a letter ready on August 9. My brother Tim also provided a brief for my appeal. Thankfully, Blue Cross relented. The redo would be covered. But there was a catch. Dr. Pendorff would have to do the surgery or he would have to decline to do it. Formally.

When we reapproached Dr. Pendorff, we told him what Steenerson proposed and what BCBS had said, and we were shocked to hear him changing his tune. Maybe he would give it a shot after all. He was annoyed that I had canceled my follow-up appointment and wanted me to come in again for another exam. We wondered if his professional competitiveness had kicked in.

Dr. Pendorff ultimately acceded to our wishes. In a phone conversation, Marty told him, flat out, that we would rather go with a practice with which we were more comfortable. In a terse letter on October 4, he told Blue Cross Blue Shield that after careful consideration, he was "not prepared to accept Mr. Holston as a surgical candidate."

The day after Thanksgiving, Marty and I drove to my pre-op appointment with Dr. Steenerson. I was on his surgical calendar for December 6. When he looked at my right ear with an otoscope, he was startled. He summoned us to another exam room that had a microscope on a sort of crane that looked like something from a dentist's office. He grumbled. Even I, unable to hear, could tell by his expression that something wasn't right.

He told Marty that the electrode array of my implant was "extruded." It had somehow worked its way through the tissue. A portion of it was visible, even to the naked eye, in my ear canal. Viewed through the microscope, he said he could actually see the tiny transistor along the wire. And to make matters worse, my eardrum appeared to have detached since he had last seen me.

He put my surgery on hold, told me to avoid showering until I could get an earplug that would seal it, and sent me home. Marty and I didn't talk much on the drive back to Athens. We were both at a loss for words, not that I would have been able to understand much of hers anyway.

A few days later, Dr. Steenerson himself called. He told Marty he had no other choice but to cancel my December 6 surgery. He said that the extrusion and the damage in my ear canal would make what already promised to be a long, tricky operation longer and trickier. He said that it would likely take six or seven hours and that, at his age, seventy, he was concerned about having the stamina and acuity to do the operation properly.

Just before Christmas, we visited my Aunt Nell in Mississippi. On the return trip, we swung south through Mobile to see my brother and his family and to have him see if he could tweak the setting on my left-ear hearing aid. I was starting to see it as my best hope.

At the hearing clinic he oversaw at the University of South Alabama, he introduced me to the new ENT on staff, a doctor with a name like a *Smokey and the Bandit* character: Wylie Justice.

Tim had already been talking to him about my case, and Dr. Justice was eager to see this unusual malfunction in person. He had me lie down on an exam table, aimed the microscope at my right ear, and had me look at the monitor on the other side of the room. And there it was, just as Steenerson had described. It looked like a lonesome loop of Christmas lights hanging from the eaves of a house.

Dr. Justice said the urgency of the revision surgery was greater than ever. I was at risk for all manner of infections. His advice was that I go to the House Ear Institute in Los Angeles.

Neither Marty nor I had heard of it. Dr. Justice said that House is to ear problems what the MD Anderson Clinic in Houston is to cancer treatment and research. It was founded by an otologist who was a pioneer in hearing-restoration surgeries. Dr. Justice said the House clinic was internationally renowned, the sort of place Swiss bankers and Saudi oil sheikhs jet to when they have serious hearing problems. He urged us to contact the clinic as soon as we got back to Athens.

Chapter 27

House Call

We took Dr. Justice at his word. Once we were home, we unloaded the car, let the cats out to play, and then went online looking for information about the House Institute. The photos on its website were impressive, the building all gleaming chrome and glass with a beautiful fountain out front. The website's history section said that physicians and scientists at the institute founded by Dr. Howard P. House had developed and perfected the cochlear implant and auditory brain stem implant for patients who are totally deaf. It listed ten ear specialists on staff, seven of whom performed surgeries.

On the second day of January, Marty phoned the House Institute's main number and asked to be transferred to someone she could talk to about a cochlear implant revision surgery. She was connected to Dawna Mills, a doctor of audiology. After listening to Marty recap my cochlear misadventure, Mills said we should send them my records and most recent CT scan as soon as we could gather all the materials.

We priority-mailed the records two days later. We waited, but I didn't just sit around twiddling my thumbs or tugging on my ear lobes. By this time, I had started to learn "speechreading"—a skill formerly known as lipreading—at the University of Georgia's

Department of Speech and Hearing. Twice a week, I would go to a booth at the department, and a young woman who was finishing up her masters, Kristina Kishimoto, would coach me on how the mouth forms various vowels and consonants, and she would read to me, sans hearing aid and implant, from a *Time* magazine or a Tom Clancy novel. My task was to answer her questions about what she'd read, or to recap.

I was not surprised to find that I was lousy at it. My brother told me that even after three decades in audiology, he had never gotten very good at it. Not only is it an inexact art, he said, but some people just have more of a knack for it than others. Obviously, neither of us had gotten the speechreading gene.

Still, I tried. I felt as though I needed every tool in my belt that I could acquire. Putting Kristina's lessons into practice, however, was easier said than done. I quickly came to understand that people often don't continue to face you when they're speaking. They cover their mouths, they look away, they mumble. Even Marty had to be reminded that she had to look at me when she talked. I also realized how much I had come to reflexively avoid conversation at work. I still tended to email colleagues, even those whose offices are only a few steps from mine. I made a mental note: Stop that! Reengage.

On the morning of February 8, I opened my email files at work and saw that I had a message from the House Institute. It was from a William Slattery, one of the surgeons.

"It currently appears upon reviewing your CT scan that the cochlear implant is coming out of the ear and it has actually extended through the ear canal and through the eardrum," Dr. Slattery wrote, his words metaphorical music to my ears. "I do have experience with this kind of case. I would suggest that you have revision surgery.

"I would be happy to set this up if you like," he continued. "To do this I would close off your ear canal, which would not be a significant deformity. At the same time, I would go ahead and put in a new cochlear implant. I think this would help you significantly. If you decide that you want to move forward with this or if you want to discuss it further, please let me know."

I texted Marty within seconds: "Just heard from a doctor at House Institute. He says he can do the do-over. Makes it sound like a piece of cake."

She texted back: "Come home!"

I locked up my office, told the receptionist I was leaving, raced to the parking deck, and did my best not to speed on the way home. Marty was waiting at the front door to embrace me. She was aglow—happier even than I was. We went out to dinner to celebrate.

Back home, just after nine o'clock, Marty answered a telephone call. She saw me looking her way quizzically and mouthed, "It's Slattery," as she jabbed her finger at the phone. He had some questions for me that she excitedly scribbled on a pad. I filled in some history for him, and she took down the name and number of an associate of his he wanted us to contact. "He sounds confident and really nice," she said when the House call ended. She made two fists in front of her chest and did a happy dance.

*   *   *

At my speechreading session with Kristina a couple of days later, her boss, Dr. Holly Kaplan, dropped by to see how it was going. I told her I thought I was getting a little better at it, and Kristina concurred. I also told her that I had heard back from House and that one of the surgeons there believed he could repair the damage.

"Who's the doctor?" she asked.

"A guy name William Slattery," I said.

"Slattery,'" she repeated, her eyes widening.

I felt as if I were in the scene from *Bye Bye Birdie* when Kim's family learns they're going to be on Ed Sullivan's TV variety show.

Celestial beams of light shine upon them. *"Ed Sul-li-van!!"* they sing as one, starry-eyed and reverent.

"You've heard of him?" I asked.

"Oh, my," she said. "He's only, like, one of the best three or four cochlear surgeons in the world."

Bill Slat-ter-y!!

I began to think my prospects were looking up.

Chapter 28

Crossed Swords

D r. Steenerson graciously signed off on the plan to have Dr. Slattery rewire me. But Blue Cross Blue Shield of Georgia, true to form, balked. Bad enough that I couldn't find a surgeon on its roster, but did I really have to go to California? Hey, why not London? Zurich? Give these hypochondriacs an inch . . .

But I persisted. And Marty, my self-proclaimed personal assistant and squeaky wheel, *really* persisted. And with Hoffmann, Steenerson, Weber, and Slattery, plus my brother the audiology professor, my dentist, and my yard guy backing me up, BCBS relented and said, "Go West, old man."

Marty immediately began looking online for affordable flights from Atlanta to Los Angeles in April, the soonest Dr. Slattery could get me on his schedule. From speaking with Slattery's associate, she learned, much to our relief, that House Institute patients were eligible to stay in budget-rate accommodations nearby. Our house was buzzing with anticipation.

But life, we were soon reminded, doesn't necessarily deal you one challenge at a time. Just because you lose your hearing or have to have breast-cancer surgery, that doesn't mean you get a pass on everything else.

In early March, Marty learned that her father's heart was failing and that his doctor in Nebraska was sending him to Kansas City for surgery. Don had already had a bypass, and this new surgery was his best hope of surviving. Marty flew out—not to be with her dad, but to watch over her mom in his stead at their house in tiny Denton, Nebraska.

Marty kept me up to date via text and the CapTel phone. The news was not good. Her father's heart tissue was too soft for the operation. The surgeon sewed him back up and sent him to ICU. "What a perfect metaphor for my dad," Marty texted me. "Outwardly tough, inwardly mushy."

Her sister Margaret came to relieve her in Denton, and she moved on to her sister Amy's house in Omaha, from where she was scheduled to fly home. There was no time for her to drive to Kansas City, but she did get to talk to her father on the phone. Early on the morning of her flight, her niece, a nurse at the hospital in Kansas City, phoned to tell Marty and Amy their father had passed on.

I picked Marty up at the Atlanta airport. As we drove home, she told me about seeing formations of migrating geese during her sunrise walk and about the empty seat next to her on her otherwise packed plane. She considered both signs from her dad, Don. She said little else. It was late when we got to our house. We were both so exhausted, we left her bags in the car.

Early in the morning, before dawn, Marty, with her wildcat ears, heard something.

When she came downstairs and parted the front drapes, she saw that the interior light was on in my car. Then she realized there was a white truck idling near it. She slipped on shoes, wrapped her jangle of keys around her fist, and charged out across the front porch yelling. The would-be burglar jumped in his truck and sped off.

Already angry and sad about her father, now she was furious. She ran to the street but couldn't see the intruder's license plate. She dialed 911. A squad car arrived in minutes. The police dusted my car for prints and took notes about the truck and what she'd seen and what she'd done.

I slept through it all. Still in her pajamas, she woke me and told me about the car. She also told me one of the officers had said, "You mentioned your husband. Is he not here?"

She said she told him, "No, he's here. He's deaf. World War III could break out in our living room and he wouldn't know."

According to Marty, the cop said, "Wow. You're kind of a badass." I saw her smile for the first time since I met her at the airport.

Preparing for our trip to Los Angeles—packing and arranging for neighbors to tend to our herd of cats—provided a needed distraction. Hope and anticipation offset grief. We flew from Atlanta to Los Angeles on April 14, a Sunday. Dr. Slattery and his staff created a schedule for us that minimized what was going to be a costly stay under any circumstances. The plan was that I would do my pre-op on Monday, have surgery on Tuesday, rest on Wednesday and Thursday, have my post-op appointment on Friday, and fly home on Saturday.

We had decided to make a sort of vacation of it: see some sights, get my head stroked and bored like the Beach Boys' little deuce coupe, see some more sights if possible, and fly home to heal.

Flying in on a Sunday, early, was wise. Sundays are as quiet as Los Angeles gets, and the last thing we wanted was the stress of driving in multilane freeway traffic while looking for exits whose whereabouts I could only guess at. In all my trips to LA for TV-related events over the years, I had driven as little as I could get away with for that very reason. Miss an exit, and before you know it, you're in Petaluma. I was once an hour late for an interview appointment with William Peterson, the star of *CSI,* because I saw my freeway exit too late. But this time, it was quiet. There was time to look and anticipate. Plus, we had a GPS, the greatest boon to travel since trail mix. We found St. Vincent's so easily, it was as if we had a programmed\self-driving car.

The House Ear Institute sits just across the street from St. Vincent Medical Center, the oldest hospital in Los Angeles. Just a couple of blocks away, on Wilshire Boulevard, is an entrance to Macarthur Park, immortalized in Jimmy Webb's much-recorded song about a shattered love affair and cake left out in the rain. The hospital was founded as the Los Angeles Infirmary in 1856 by the Daughters of Charity of St. Vincent de Paul, an order of nuns. Seton Hall, the nuns' quarters, still sits on the site, shadowed by the now huge, high-rise hospital. Half of Seton Hall's rooms have been converted into a sort of hospice/motel, with spartan but comfortable suites, complete with kitchenettes, where patients can stay for about the same rate as an Embassy Suites. An Embassy Suites in Omaha or Baton Rouge, that is, not Los Angeles. In other words, the rates are ridiculously, beatifically reasonable.

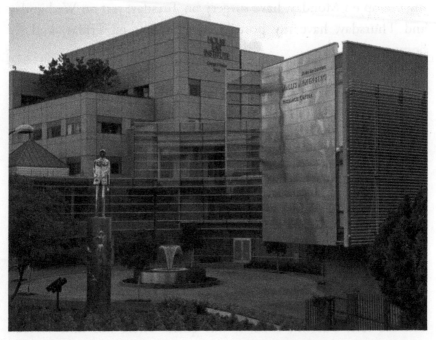

Courtesy of the House Ear Institute

We checked in and surveyed our room. The exterior wall was all window and unobstructed, affording us a panoramic view of tiled rooftops, palm-tree greenery, and a rise of mountains in the distance. We decided to spend the afternoon exploring the hilly neighborhood with its world bazaar of shops and babel of signage. We ate dinner at a Peruvian café where Marty's modest knowledge of Spanish was enough to get us a great meal and royal treatment.

The next morning, we walked across the street from Seton Hall to the House Institute. It was as Oz-like as the online photos we'd seen had suggested, all glass and gleaming chrome. In a garden to the left of the entrance, a life-sized sculpture, a silvery figure on a tall pedestal, loomed against the blue sky like a Tin Man in a lab coat. The near side of the pedestal was embossed with the figure of a man reaching up with his right hand, his left pressed to his ear. In the lobby was a model of the human ear the size of a children's playground slide. We stopped to shoot a few photos with our phones and then checked in.

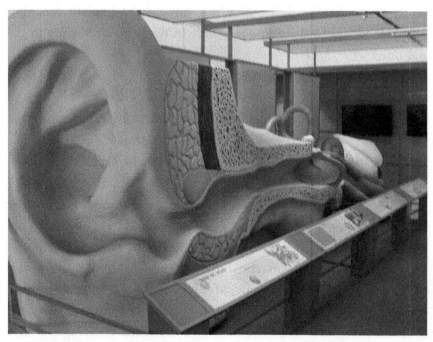

Courtesy of the House Ear Institute

Once my name was called, we were sent to an exam room down a long hall and waited. With Holly Kaplan's admiring "Slattery" echoing through my head, I halfway expected him to come flying in with a cape billowing behind. But when he turned up, William Slattery wore a standard white lab coat over a white shirt and gray suit pants. He was handsome in a soft, unassuming way and, like so many creatures of the medical world, pale. His manner was, likewise, unpretentious and pleasant—none of that godlike arrogance. He told us that while he had performed hundreds of revision surgeries, redos were actually quite rare in the larger scheme.

He went over my medical history and explained what he planned to do and why he believed he could make a more effective placement of the electrode array. He declined, even when directly asked, to critique the original operation, other than to acknowledge that the array had indeed migrated.

The only surprise for us—and the only thing to give me a little pause—was that he didn't like how my current implant was situated. He would be drilling a new hole in my head and filling in the old one.

"Plastic Wood?" I jested.

The surgeon laughed. No, a kind of bone paste.

He also explained that he would have to surgically restore the tissue in my ear canal and build a sort of dermatological manhole cover over it to keep water from leaking past the detached eardrum and into my head.

Marty and I decided to make the most of the rest of the day. We set the GPS for Santa Monica. The sun was out, the weather mild, and we wanted to see some ocean before I went under the knife.

After we walked on the beach at Santa Monica, we drove north up the coastal highway through Malibu. We stumbled onto Pepperdine University, famous for its water polo team and partying, perched on a grassy slope overlooking the Pacific. Heading east into the mountains behind the school, we found ourselves on a snaking, spiraling highway that felt as though it were unspooling before us. It was like being inside a cochlea. We considered it a good sign.

Chapter 29

Ear We Go Again

Early Tuesday morning, sleepy-eyed and wishing I could have my usual dose of caffeine, I made the short walk from Seton Hall to St. Vincent's, holding hands with Marty. We had talked about the possibility that a new implant might not work any better than the original. We had talked about the possibility that the removal of the old array might damage my ear so badly that I would have no hearing at all.

"There's always ASL," Marty said.

I laughed, and it wasn't just nervous laughter. I was an old hand at this. Or an old ear, as it were. I was grateful we didn't have to drive half asleep on an unfamiliar freeway, as we'd done in Atlanta. I could simply stroll. There was a garden in bloom. I hadn't shaved my head, knowing this time that the prep nurse would merely buzz away a strip of gray hair just above my right ear. When the orderly rolled my gurney toward the operating room, it was down a long, glassed-in corridor, not the beige hallway of Atlanta. I could see fronds of palm trees flitting by. I could see blue sky. It was like riding an elevated monorail at Disney World. It was like a vacation. The drugs had obviously kicked in.

I have only the vaguest recollection of the OR. The lights were very bright. I was lifted off the gurney and onto the operating table.

The surgery took six hours. My first wake-up memory is of Marty trying to get me to eat something. I was a slug. I had no appetite. I was doing well to eat ice chips.

She kept insisting. "They're not going to let you go until you eat," she said, holding out a plastic cup of apple sauce. "Eat. Come on, baby. Eat. I'm ready to get us out of here."

After forty minutes or so, a male nurse transferred me to a wheelchair and took us on what seemed like an endless, labyrinthine trip through the bowels of St. Vincent's and back to our room at Seton Hall. I crawled into bed and slept like a stone until the next morning.

I awoke feeling . . . good. For someone who'd just had one hole bored in his skull and another one filled, I felt shockingly normal. I've felt worse in the morning after a couple of martinis. Marty snapped some pictures of me with my black eye and bulging head bandage while I savored a cup of coffee. I put a plastic cap over my head and got into the shower.

When I came out of the bathroom, she greeted me with a curlicue mustache she'd made by peeling an orange in one continuous loop. She looked like a cross between Salvador Dalí and a ray of sunshine. I laughed harder than I had laughed in a long time.

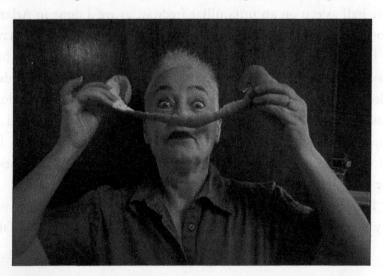

Then we went to breakfast. We walked to the hospital's cafeteria. After she had polished off a plate of eggs and sausage, Marty spotted an old upright piano against the wall. While I savored my own plate of cholesterol, she flipped the piano open, tested it, ascertained it was pretty much in tune, and sat down to play. I couldn't hear a note, but I could see hospital staff and other patients paying attention. I saw hands applauding. Magic moments were piling up. I was feeling optimistic.

For our noonday meal, Marty suggested El Pollo Loco, which we had passed during our presurgery exploration of the neighborhood. "I don't know," I said. "That sidewalk is pretty steep."

"I'll have your arm," she said. "It just smells sooo good."

Chapter 30

I Love LA

The El Pollo Loco sits a block and a half down the western slope of Alvarado Street from St. Vincent's. We made it down the hill without me falling. Marty ordered for us—grilled chicken with sweet plantains and a bowl of rice and beans. The air was pungent and steamy with the scent of lime, cumin, garlic, and onion. The noonday rush was on. To minimize the clamor for her, we stationed ourselves at a small table behind an under-glass condiment buffet stocked with a luscious array of salsas and peppers.

From my window-facing seat, I had a broad view of diversity on parade. Across Alvarado I could see a small shop that sells knockoff Major League Baseball caps and Chinese porn DVDs, a Guatemalan café, and a vegetable stand-cum-smoothie parlor run by a refugee from Senegal. The diners at El Pollo Loco represented probably half the countries of Central America and several African nations, as well. We were two of the paler faces in sight.

I had on beat-up old blue jeans with big, ravel-fringed holes in the knees, grubby tennis shoes, and a lime-colored hoodie two sizes too small for me. I'd had to borrow it from Marty because I hadn't packed warm clothes for an unexpectedly chilly Southern California spring. I hadn't shaved or washed my hair for three days. I had a black eye and a swollen cheek on the right side. I looked as though I should have a grocery cart overflowing with ragged clothes and

bulging plastic trash bags parked outside. Wrapped around my head
was a white bandage that included a mound of gauze the size of a
C-cup bra over my right ear.

As we waited for our number to be called, a man in a blue
T-shirt with a stack of pamphlets in his hand and a bundle of
what appeared to be multicolored shoelaces slung over his shoulder
greeted my wife in Mexican-accented English and asked if she'd like
to make a donation to his church. Marty lived in New York City
for seven years. She is pretty much immune to the pleas of street
preachers, vendors, hustlers, and panhandlers. She shook her head
and said quietly and politely, "No, thank you."

The man started to walk away, then turned back toward us.

"Did he just get out of the hospital?" he asked, glancing at me.

"Yes," my wife answered.

He leaned in closer. "Does he need a place to stay?"

"No, thank you," she said.

As the man moved to the next table and hit up another customer, this time speaking Spanish, my wife turned to me smiling
and rolling her eyes.

I hadn't actually *heard* any of this, of course. Marty recapped
the exchange later, using a combination of slowly spoken words,
scribbles on a steno pad, and pantomime.

And then I laughed out loud. I knew that I had laughed because
I could feel it in my throat and chest. I was back where I started
three years earlier: functionally deaf.

Lunch at the crazy chicken joint marked the beginning of the
second half of the best vacation I ever had that encompassed anesthesia, scalpels, and power tools.

On Thursday, I was feeling sturdy enough for us to spend a
good portion of the day touring an exhibit of German Expressionist
art at the Los Angeles County Museum of Art (LACMA). Marty
drove. I wasn't feeling quite that clearheaded yet.

Even though I hid the white bandage under one of Marty's floral scarves, I was still a little anxious about the prospect of being gaped at, but my self-consciousness was unfounded. I hadn't factored in that this was Los Angeles, where exotic headgear—here a beret, there a turban, there a hijab—is hardly a rare sight. What was one more guy with a do-rag?

On the drive back to Seton Hall, Marty pulled to the curb several times to let me hop out and snap photos. We had discovered earlier in the week that the Westlake area of Los Angeles has an abundance of wonderful antique signage, relics of the twenties and thirties, for someone who has an eye fresh enough to notice.

That evening, we had dinner at an outdoor restaurant in the Farmers Market. On Friday night, we explored Koreatown, randomly choosing one of the many small cafés. The menu was entirely in Korean, and the waitress spoke about ten words of English. We accidentally ordered enough food for five or six people to feast on, including a couple of dishes that looked like something Dr. Seuss dreamed up. It was incredible.

We had already taken care of the only remaining business earlier in the day: a check-out appointment with Dr. Slattery. He was happy with the incision, happy with the sutures where he'd sewn my outer ear back to my head, and happy with the cap he'd created to block off my ear canal. He alerted us that my ear might bleed on the next day's flight back to Georgia because of cabin pressure changes, but he said it was nothing to worry about. I made a note to have a pocketful of tissues.

I didn't need them. The flight was uneventful. Likewise the drive from Atlanta to Athens. I slept soundly (and soundless) in my own bed that night, aided by a dose of Vicodin. On Sunday, the wait began. Until implant activation number two, I would have only the limited, Widex-assisted hearing in my left ear.

Chapter 31

Reactivation

My activation was scheduled for Monday, April 29, less than two weeks after my surgery. The first time around, the wait had been six weeks. Dr. Slattery was confident that I would be ready sooner this time. He had also graciously deferred to Dr. Steenerson in Atlanta so that I wouldn't have to fly back to Los Angeles just to have the incision checked. That Sunday night, I slept little. If anything, the second time around was scarier. In the fall of 2010, I had been wildly hopeful, my expectations boosted by what every medical professional I'd dealt with, including my own brother, had said about what a great implant candidate I was. Now, I was, if not a battered veteran, a bruised orange.

I tamped down my hopes. My hearing with the new implant could be better or about the same. Or worse. By this time, I not only had the benefit of experience, but I had also discovered a US Food and Drug Administration website, www.fda.gov (see Appendix, page 203), that had sections explaining the possible benefits and risks of a wide variety of medical devices, including cochlear implants. It had all the unsentimental, objective, nonpromotional information that I'd had difficulty finding when I was considering an implant the first time.

What I did know for sure was that the California expedition had been worthwhile even if Dr. Slattery's efforts were in vain. With

Marty's help, I had negotiated a huge, complex city I had found intimidating even in the years when I had full hearing. I not only had come to realize there was indeed a book to emerge from all this monkey business, but I also had a brainstorm, an idea for another artistic project, a photo book.

Most important of all, I had met other House Institute patients at the Seton Hall dormitory, including a Vietnam veteran whose decades of combat-related deafness was belatedly corrected by House doctors and a family from Canada whose daughter was undergoing experimental treatment for hereditary, potentially fatal inner-ear tumors. They gave me even more perspective on my modest problem.

On that sunny April morning, we made the ninety-minute drive from Athens to Dr. Steenerson's office in northwest Atlanta. He removed the stitches around my ear, cleaned up the incision, and examined my ear canal. He seemed a little disappointed that Dr. Slattery had not chosen to employ the complicated "back-door" maneuver that he had planned to undertake, but he spoke admiringly of the other surgeon's work.

He sent us down the hall to Cindy Gary's office for the activation. Atop my reddened, right ear she placed a gunmetal-gray Cochlear Americas New Freedom processor, the model to which the company had reverted after the Nucleus 5 recall. From the processor trailed a thin electrical cord that was plugged into her laptop. She attached the magnetized connection to the tiny steel chip embedded in my skull. I braced for the big turn-on. I knew not to expect more clarity immediately. I had been bionic for more than two years, but this was a different electrode array differently placed, not to mention a different processor. What I got when Cindy threw the switch was surprising—far better than the shzzzzzz chzzzzzzt tssss chvzzzzr of the 2010 activation—but a long way from clear.

I could almost make out words she spoke, but they seemed to be at the very bottom of the sound mix, overwhelmed by a reverberating echo that made my head hurt. Even when she toned down the reverb, words sounded distorted, as if they had audio tails trailing behind them. It made me think of a train engine-shaped wooden toy one of my kids had years back. When you blew into it, it approximated the toots of a steam locomotive. On the drive home, Marty's attempts to talk to me sounded like a choo-choo. We tabled the conversation until later. She turned on NPR. I listened to the whistling sound of the tires on asphalt.

Once again, I was advised not to use my left-ear hearing aid for a month, except in case of emergency. By the second day, I was wondering if dinner qualified. We had house guests, two young actors from Atlanta who were in rehearsals for a production at Rose of Athens, a theater company for which Marty composes. They're quick, witty conversationalists we'd known for several years, but they might as well have been pantomiming Punch and Judy puppets for all I could discern. Even with intense concentration, it was hard to make out more than an occasional word. Sound in my implant ear was watery, wheezy, and so seemingly loud that it masked the little bit of hearing I had in my unaided left.

Next morning, when they'd all gone to the theater, I fired up Cochlear America's Sound and Way Beyond program on my laptop. Time to get back on the horse, I told myself. This is rehab. This is audio calisthenics.

My scores were lower than those of my first tries two years before. On vowel recognition, I got only eleven out of forty-eight utterances correct.

On May 10, we went back to the Atlanta Ear Clinic for another mapping session with Cindy Gary. This time, there was a definite uptick. At the end of the tweaking, we had a fifteen-minute conversation about the Diego Rivera-Freida Kahlo exhibit at Atlanta's High Museum, which Marty and I had recently toured. It was animated and lively. And even with Cindy speaking with her mouth hidden behind a hand-held screen, I understood about 90 percent of her comments and questions. She said it was the best conversation we'd had in the more than two years I'd been a client. I felt like a kindergartner getting a gold star.

The timing couldn't have better. On May 16, a Thursday, I had to fly to New York to do my part in staging the Peabody Awards ceremony at the Waldorf-Astoria Hotel. And I was flying unaccompanied. Marty's Rose of Athens show wouldn't close until Friday night. She would fly up on Saturday afternoon to join me.

The show was an adaption of Roald Dahl's children's book, *James and the Giant Peach*, for which she had composed original songs. I contributed one as well, the only song I had written since my hearing and pitch degraded.

Inspired by the orphaned hero's vigils from the gables of his gruesome guardians' Victorian house, it was titled "I Can See Home."

If I climb way up on the rickety roof
Crane my neck and strain my eyes
In my I mind I'm sure that I can see
The place that my heart desires

I can see home/On the horizon
I can see home/In my mind's eye
I can see home/Wish I could fly by
I can see home/I can see home

I couldn't quite identify with James's adventure inside a huge, fuzzy fruit, but his yearning? I knew that only too well.

* * *

When I boarded my New York flight in Atlanta, my hearing was the sharpest it had been in years. When I landed at LaGuardia, not so sharp, and no idea why. Fatigue. Cabin pressure changes. The salty complimentary pretzels.

Luckily, the routine was familiar. I got in line and got loaded into a taxi. I could barely understand the driver, but hey, it's New York City, what else is new? The driver and I managed. I checked in at the Waldorf, texted Marty that I had arrived, placed both my hearing devices on the nightstand—"radio silence," I call it—and took a nap. I dined alone at Cafe Metro, a deli a couple of blocks from the hotel. I had to have the cashier show me the receipt because I couldn't understand the total she spoke. I fell asleep later watching *Game of Thrones* reruns on HBO. I wondered how the Lannisters and Starks dealt with the deaf. Did they feed them to the dragons?

Our traditional Friday morning meeting with the hotel staff—the event manager, florist, head electrician, et al., seated on one side of a long table and we Peabody folk seated on the other, like facing the Last Supper tableaux—was another silent movie for me to smile and nod through. I realized I had come to pride myself in being able to fake hearing and engagement. At least I thought I was pulling it off.

After we got our temporary Peabody office set up in the hotel's Cole Porter suite, I went out roaming midtown Manhattan, as always on these annual trips looking for street scenes and architectural novelties to photograph. I had to cut the photo safari short. Even with my newly mapped implant geared down to the lowest volume setting, the roar and screech of the city on a Friday afternoon was cataclysmic. And silent running was not an option, not with traffic as frantic as it was. I remembered a time when I was driving in the city during my *Newsday* tenure and almost hit a distracted pedestrian, who turned out to be Neil Simon. He shook his fist at me.

I was more than distracted. I was nervous. I retreated to my cave at the hotel with a fresh copy of the *New Yorker*.

Saturday was quieter. Fewer people on the streets. An almost leisurely feel to the East Side of midtown. I hiked all the way up to Central Park. Later that evening, I curled up on a sofa in my room, found a basketball game on TV, and set my cell phone beside me. I turned off my hearing devices to rest my ears. I had texted Marty the room number. She would text me when she got to the Waldorf.

When I awoke, I noticed the little red light on my phone was blinking. I checked the time on my cell. It was almost 1 a.m. I frantically went to my text message file and saw that I had a string of them, dating back almost an hour. The last one read, "WTF, baby? I AM OUTSIDE YOUR DOOR!!!"

I looked toward the door. It was slightly ajar, caught on the safety latch. I quickly put on my ears. Through the narrow opening, a hand protruded. Waving.

I rushed to the door and opened it to find Marty and a comparably annoyed Waldorf bellman standing a step back into the hallway. "Hey honey," I said, smiling sheepishly. Marty just gave me an evil look as she dragged her suitcase inside and flopped onto the sofa. I grabbed my wallet and gave the bellman a tip.

"What the hell were you doing?" she said after I shut the door. "You knew when I was supposed to get here! I've been skulking around the hallway for almost an hour. I think the bellhop thought I was a lady of the evening. I had to go downstairs to the front desk, get a porter, and then show an ID and confirm that I was registered to your room. We rang the phone in the room. We had to stop pounding on the door because he was afraid he was going to wake up other guests."

I had no answer.

Chapter 32
Rabbit Box

My reconditioned ears perked up when I saw that Rabbit Box, Athens's answer to the public-radio storytelling series *The Moth*, had listed "Down the Rabbit Hole" on its website as one of its forthcoming themes. In keeping with my vow to exploit my disability to positive effect whenever possible, I pitched myself via email for the June edition and got a message back telling me I would be on the bill.

I wrote, memorized, and presented the following rant/yarn at The Melting Point, the Athens music venue that hosts the monthly storytelling jams. I was one of eight performers that evening, facing double-tier seating of about 250 people.

I stepped up to the microphone in khakis, a single spotlight on me in a white dress shirt and sneakers, my script in hand. I dropped the pages to the stage and began by telling the audience that however long, convoluted, and preposterous it might seem, it was in fact like a *Reader's Digest* version, condensed and simplified and cleansed of numerous expletives:

I'm not sure how much you know about the topography of our beloved Peach state, but in addition to mountains and swamps and savanna, it has an enormous rabbit hole. Not just a single rabbit hole, either, but a warren of labyrinth-like proportions with portals in Columbus, Atlanta, and other places. It's a strange, nonsensical maze entirely worthy of Lewis Carroll and his Jabberwock and Red Queen and Tweedle Dee and Dum.

You may recognize this rabbit hole by its common name—Blue Cross Blue Shield of Georgia—or by its acronym, the very fitting BC BS.

Now, we all know that insurance companies sometimes seem to go out of their way to make transactions difficult for their clients. You can get the feeling they're hoping you'll get frustrated and give up. But I didn't truly appreciate Blue Cross Blue Shield of Georgia's Mad Hatter sensibility until I had the misfortune of waking up one morning in March 2010 to find myself, for all practical purposes, deaf.

One of those practical purposes was communicating by telephone. After trying various drugs and therapies, the ear specialist I was seeing determined that a cochlear implant—a sort of bionic ear—was my only hope of hearing much again. I had to start wrangling with BCBS over coverage. They disputed whether I was deaf enough.

I couldn't phone them, so I went to their website, thinking I would start an email dialogue. But, it turned out, you can't have an email correspondence with them. You can only email to request a call back.

Which I did. And there ensued a series of conversations that went something like this.

My wife would answer the phone. A BCBS representative would say, "May I speak to Mr. Holston?" Marty would say, "I'm sorry, but Mr. Holston has lost his hearing. He can't talk on the phone. You can talk to him through me."

And the BCBS customer service rep would say, "Sorry, but you're not authorized to speak for him." And she would say, "Well, he can't hear, but he can talk. What if I write down what you need from him so he can read it and then answer you aloud?" And the rep would say, "Sorry, we can't do that."

And she would say, "Why?" And the rep would say, "How do we know it's really him?"

And Marty would say, "Well, the same way you'd have known if he had answered the phone." And they would not be amused.

She ultimately learned that I needed to fill out something called a HIPPA form that would allow her to speak for me. I would need to download the form from the website, fill it out, and fax it to a BCBS number.

I did this. And the next time BCBS called, we went through the same nutty conversation. I filled out HIPPA forms four times before they finally acknowledged Marty as my designated spokesperson. The first three forms just disappeared into the rabbit hole.

I finally had cochlear implant surgery October 2010, and BCBS, bless its little bunny heart, paid for it. And I got out of their hair, pardon the expression.

Alas, the cochlear implant was not working as it was supposed to work. By early 2011, it was pretty clear something was amiss. Both the manufacturer and my doctors recommended a do-over. I had to revisit the rabbit hole.

By this time, since I still couldn't talk on the phone, I had acquired a CapTel phone—a phone that translates the worlds of the person you call into captions you can read on a little screen. I wanted to spare my wife the frustration, so I tried calling BCBS.

Trouble was, there's a time delay on the captions. So when I didn't respond immediately to the automated systems' request for various information—punching in numbers and stuff—it would hang up on me, presuming I had lost interest or died or something.

So it was back to emails and BCBS calling my house and telling Marty it couldn't talk to her unless I filled out a HIPPA form.

I finally got my implant do-over—in April of this year. I had to go to a clinic in Los Angeles for the surgery. No surgeon in Georgia felt qualified to do it. I know this because Blue Cross insisted I see each of them and get a rejection. So, I went to California with an out-of-state, out-of-plan authorization from BCBS in hand.

But, as they say down in the rabbit hole, it gets curiouser and curiouser. A couple of weeks after my implant do-over, I start getting notices from doctors and labs saying that Blue Cross has declined to pay my claims. They include a big, big bill from the doctor in California who BCBS had authorized to do my surgery. They all wanted their money.

I used my trusty CapTel phone to call BCBS. By now I know all the codes so I don't get cut off. I finally get a human on the phone and explain what's going on. She tells me it's because I turned sixty-five in March and I'm now on Medicare. I tell her I'm not. That I am still employed by UGA and still their client. She says, well, you should have informed us. And I say, well, doesn't the fact that I'm still paying you several hundred dollars a month in premiums tell you something?

Anyway, she vows to correct the error and notify the creditors. Two weeks later, I start getting second notices. There's mention of collection agencies.

I get back on the CapTel with BCBS. An agent named Michelle is apologetic. She swears she'll straighten it out. She asks if she can put me on hold while she calls one of the creditors, LabCorp. And, once again, it gets curiouser and curiouser.

I can hear the conversation. Or, rather, I can see the captions, a few seconds behind. The two customer reps are chattering away. I see the name Michelle popping up. I politely interrupt. "Excuse me, but are you both named Michelle?" The captions indicate "yes"es.

I say, "Would you mind identifying yourselves before speaking as Michelle 1 and Michelle 2?"

One of the Michelles says, "That would be kind of awkward." And I say, "Well, not nearly as awkward as me trying to figure out which one of you is which from captions."

Michelle 1 assures me that the LabCorp bill is taken care of and that she will notify the other creditors of the Medicare mix-up. And she asks if there's anything else she can do for me.

I say, actually, yes, there is. When this call began, BCBS's automated system notified me that it was being recorded. I tell her I'm a professional journalist and that I'm writing a book about my hearing-loss adventure. I tell her it would be helpful to have that recording so I can quote everybody correctly.

After a long pause, I read the caption of her saying, "I'll see what I can do."

That was four weeks ago.

I am still waiting for my copy of the recording.

I'm not upset, though. I'm a patient man as you can see. I've retained a sense of humor about all this. And I'm an optimist.

I have every confidence that one day soon that recording will be delivered to my doorstep.

By a white rabbit.

A white rabbit wearing a waistcoat and carrying a pocket watch, a blue cross, and a blue shield.

The audience rewarded my tale with sustained, enthusiastic applause. They may have been clapping for my perseverance rather than my skill as a monologist, but whatever the case, it felt good.

Chapter 33

Back to Life

Not only was I now able to hear big noises, but, as 2013 moved into its second half, I was hearing small sounds better, as well. All the work I had previously done—the ah-bah, ah-sha practices and the speech therapy—had some carryover. My period of adjustment was shorter the second time around and my learning curve less steep. If the new implant was not the complete fix that Marty and I and the doctors had hoped for, it was unquestionably an improvement over the original.

My awareness of sound in general was the best it had been since before my hearing crash—possibly the best it had been eight or ten years before that. Hearing loss can creep up on you so slowly and stealthily, you don't even know it's happening. It not like fading sight, when print becomes obviously indecipherable. With my implant tuned to a wide-radius setting, I had little problem sensing a wider world around me. The crunch of gravel under my shoes still rang true and bracing. In summer, I could park myself in a chair on our deck and be surrounded by the insect symphonics in the woods behind our house. In fall, Marty and I would race off like tornado chasers when we saw murmurations of starlings or blackbirds developing. We'd find spots to park where the birds swirled above us like

M.C. Escher drawings come to life and enveloped us in a chirping canopy of sound.

I also began to find music to supplement the treasury in my head. By testing CDs one by one, I realized percussive music was my best bet. *Planet Drum,* an album by Grateful Dead drummer Mickey Hart, jumped to the top of my in-car Top Ten. So did a CD I picked up at a used-record store by an African percussionist named Odo Addy. I discovered I could still appreciate *Bach on Wood,* an LP of classical chestnuts played on xylophone and marimba that I'd long had. I borrowed a CD of Balinese gamelan music from the local public library and found that, in all its bonging, clanging dissonance, it sounded almost identical to what I remembered it sounding like to my natural ears. And I got a wonderful surprise when I played *Exotica,* a best-of CD by Martin Denny, a pianist-arranger whose combo's blend of light jazz and Hawaiian music from the early 1960s had been rediscovered and reclassified "lounge" in the nineties and early 2000s. My bionic ear didn't hear it true, but its kitschy amalgam of congas, bongos, vibes, piano, and jungle sounds—faux parrots, monkeys, and such—still sounded wonderful.

My ability to hear radio, a favored source of news and information, also improved, although with limits. The best place for me to listen was in the car, windows up, sitting still. Just starting the car diminished my comprehension, however, and driving, even slowly, masked more of what was being said. The problem is, like most people, I didn't typically sit still and listen intently. Listening to the radio is something we do casually, out of the "corner" of our ear, while focusing on driving. Or at home while making breakfast or sweeping or sewing. That sort of multitasking was still not an option for me.

Conversationally, I still struggled in even moderately noisy environments, and PA-amplified sound at meetings or speeches was mush to my ears. But one-on-one conversation was decidedly more comprehensible, especially in low-noise environments.

To maximize home conversation—and lessen aggravation for Marty—I finally gave in to Marty's pleas and tossed my home-decorating aesthetic to the wind. I assented to covering most of the hardwood flooring and ceramic tile in our house with thick carpet. We replaced some of the paintings and framed posters on the walls with fabric art. I did draw the line at her proposal to staple old egg cartons to the walls as makeshift sound absorbers. Utility has its limits.

I also decided that I was overdue to take a formal course in American Sign Language, as my efforts to learn on my own from a book never amounted to much. I signed up for a night course in ASL through UGA's office of continuing education.

Like so many of my attempts to mediate my hearing difficulties, the class proved to be a bemusing boon. I discovered at the introductory class meeting that I was the only pupil who couldn't hear well, not to mention being more than twice the age of the next-oldest students. Most were enrolled because they had aspirations to be interpreters. When the teacher on the first night surveyed us about our goals for the course—I had to have him come over and repeat the question for me—I pointed out my hearing devices and explained that my main objective was to stop driving my wife crazy.

The course almost drove me up the wall. With my implant's radius of hearing only a few feet, I often had difficulty understanding what the teacher said, and my classmates might as well have been mimes. The illustrations in the designated textbook were sometimes hard to decipher, and the demonstrations of various signs in the accompanying DVD were flashed so quickly, the way a lifelong, deaf signer would, that I would have to pause it and click through the signing frame by frame to make sense of them. One of the first words we learned to sign in class was "slow." I found myself making the sign for "slow" at my TV set. Among other gestures.

The book's authors also had some odd priorities. Its cartoon-like drawings demonstrated how I would sign "She's an expert surfer,"

"He's crazy about betting on the horses," and "Have you ever been in an earthquake?" I searched in vain for illustrations of how to sign everyday essentials such as "lawn," "pillow," or "groceries."

Still, the ASL course imposed a discipline on me—and on Marty, who practiced with me daily. Once we had gotten down basic phrases—like "Toilet, where?" and "Hungry, you?"—and gotten accustomed to ASL's unique syntax, we expanded our vocabulary with the help of a different, more diverse book titled *The Joy of Signing.* It was a big help, especially on mornings when my implant was inexplicably less effective. Plus, we learned profane signs from the Internet, great for arguments and any number of everyday frustrations.

And in the spirit of leaving no option unexplored, I looked into a newly available Bluetooth microphone, manufactured by ReSound, that was compatible with that company's hearing aids and with Cochlear Americas implants. Cochlear Americas implant kits include a small mic, about the size of a thimble, on a three-foot wire. The other end has a prong meant to be plugged into a jack in the sound processor that sits on your pinna. Its purpose is to allow the person holding the mic to speak directly to the person with the processor, minimizing background sound in, say, a restaurant or at a ball game. I had such poor comprehension with my original implant that the microphone on the wire was next to useless. When I tried again after my revision surgery, I had better luck, but there was still the matter of being tethered to whoever was holding the mic. It made me feel rather like a dog on a leash, and a spontaneous move by either party could jerk my implant right off the side of my head.

The ReSound mic, a wireless device, promised greater freedom, if nothing else. We had my cochlear audiologist, Cindy Gary, order one for me. When she taught me how to "pair" it with my processor and we began to practice, it was a revelation. Not only could I understand her almost as clearly as I could while conversing with her face-to-face from three feet away, but I still could understand when I moved out into the hallway, twenty to twenty-five feet away.

On the drive home, Marty clipped the wireless mic to her seat belt, up near her chin, and we had what was for me the most intelligible conversation we'd had in a car in three years. Road noise typically masks so many words that we had often just given up and ridden in silence.

We were having such a carefree give-and-take that we were distracted when we pulled up in front of our house at twilight. The rain we'd been trying to outrun started. Marty opened her door and popped her seat belt loose, spontaneously planning to make a run for our front porch. As the seat belt snappily retracted, it slingshot the Bluetooth out of the open door and into the downpour and the dark.

Marty dashed to the house to grab an umbrella and a flashlight. I put the car in park where it sat idling, worried that I might back over my new toy. We quickly determined the mic was not in the gutter. Beyond the gutter was the expanse of English ivy that borders our front lawn. Marty held the umbrella over us while I, flashlight clenched between my teeth, crawled on my hands and knees, pulling apart the tangles of ivy and trying to spot a black Bluetooth about the size of a matchbook.

Ten minutes and a thorough soaking later, we found it, and it wasn't short-circuited by the rain. When I pulled it from between a cluster of ivy roots, I could hear it scrape—directly in my ear.

From then on, I guarded my Bluetooth as though it were a money clip.

Chapter 34
Duluth

U nderlying the friction Marty and I had experienced after my hearing crashed was a simple reality: we spent too much time together—"joined at the hip," as she put it. Everywhere she had lived, she had friends she could confide in. And I, like my father—and, apparently, like far too many men—invested almost exclusively in my wife. Our therapist agreed. We didn't need to separate, we just needed some separate-ness.

And lo and behold, out of the Northern Lights appeared a sign.

One of the choreographers Marty had worked with at the Minneapolis Fringe Festival, Rebecca Katz, was on the faculty at the University of Minnesota-Duluth. Just after Thanksgiving, she invited Marty to be an artist-in-residence. Rebecca would create one ballet around "Duluth," a sort of new-age piano piece that Marty had composed, and another based on "Migration," a prose poem inspired by flying Vs of geese Marty had seen the previous spring, the morning her father had passed away.

Marty would be away for almost a month. In Duluth. In February. We had bid farewell to Minneapolis in 2001 largely because of our increasing intolerance of frigidity. Her willingness to go even farther north, to the icy north shore of Lake Superior no less, underscored not only her eagerness to pursue a deeply personal creative project, but also how badly we needed a break from each other.

On the first of February, I saw her off on a flight from Atlanta and returned to a house empty save for our three cats.

I had plenty to keep me occupied during the day, February being the beginning of the build-up to the Peabody Awards ceremony in May. And I relished my nighttime plans to catch up on movies Marty wasn't keen on watching—horror flicks, superhero junk, violent crime dramas like *The Departed* and *Pulp Fiction,* and old westerns with Jimmy Stewart and Randolph Scott I had seen as a kid and wondered if they held up. I really appreciated *Ride Lonesome.*

Not only did I make a concerted effort to not simply hole up with a stack of DVDs and binge-watch my way through the month, but I also made dinner dates with friends, hit the local museums and galleries, and went *out* to the movies.

I arranged for my stepdaughter to come by once a week to check phone messages and tell me if I needed to call back with my CapTel. I made a similar arrangement with one of our nearby neighbors.

Marty and I mostly kept in touch by text and email, but we made a point of not overmonitoring. I mean, what could happen?

What, indeed. First, in the second week of the month, Athens was hit by a rare ice storm. There were limbs and whole trees down all over the county, and the hilly city's famously steep streets were a slip-and-slide thrill ride for those who ventured out.

And then, well, when I got up the morning of February 15 and checked my phone, there was a text from Marty: "Are you OK? How bad was the earthquake?"

Earthquake? I logged on to my computer and called up the *Athens Banner Herald* web page. Sure enough, at about 10:30 the night before, soon after Marty and I had exchanged Valentine's Day sweet talk and I had gone to sleep, north Georgia, including Athens, had experienced a rare quake, 4.1 on the Richter scale.

After I had surveyed the house, I phoned Marty on the CapTel and told her except for the cats being unusually jumpy, everything seemed to be all right. The house wasn't tilted any worse than usual, and no vases or curios had danced off their shelves as far as I could tell. After we ended the call, I pulled out the textbook from my ASL class and found the illustration for how to sign "Have you ever been in an earthquake?"

On February 22, I got an email from Marty in which she raved about another artist-in-residence, a tap dancer from New York. I felt more than a twinge of jealousy. But she ended the email by saying, "I cannot WAIT to walk in the warmth with you. You make time for your lovely wife on Tuesday morning, ok? Maybe even go into work late? Hmmmmm? That would be nice. Loving the work. Past ready to be home."

I submitted a request the next morning for two days of vacation time.

Epilogue

To paraphrase a Grateful Dead song, what a weird, circuitous journey this turned out to be.

My loss of hearing and efforts to recover as much of it as I could—all this monkey business—have been a profound learning experience, like nothing else in my life except perhaps becoming a parent.

The first lesson I would share is that you, starting right now, should protect your ears like the precious, miraculous organs they are. Be unstintingly careful about the headphones you put over your ears and the earbuds you put in them; and use plugs at sports arenas, music clubs, and rallies and when out mowing the lawn or using a leaf blower. Don't fire a weapon without ear protection. Don't even vacuum the living room. There's no guarantee that your hearing won't fail someday for other reasons, as mine did, but it's stupid to worsen your odds. Noise isn't the only culprit we face, but it's cochlear enemy number one.

Whether you have a cochlear implant or just a hearing aid, kick your vanity to the curb. It's true that some people may see you as diminished and some may think you're less intelligent than you are, but far more will appreciate your honesty, respect your disability, and try to help you communicate. Shyness is likewise a characteristic you can't afford. If you have trouble understanding a cashier at the drugstore or a sales rep at Best Buy or Old Navy, be proactive, tell them you have challenged ears. Tell them without apology. Make light of it if you have to—even point to your device(s). It's better to be up-front.

If you find yourself longing to hear clear, effortlessly comprehensible sounds, remember you have other senses and that most likely you take them for granted, too. Make a point of paying more attention to your senses of touch, taste, and smell, not just for compensation, but for stimulation. And if you still have vision, look closely. There's so much more to see.

Nobody's perfect. We're all impaired, some way or other. It's our natural state. Hearing loss is just one more limit we have to work around.

Maintaining a sense of humor is crucial. I know, I know. Going deaf isn't funny. Except when it is.

Recognize that while the cochlear implant is a technological marvel, it isn't foolproof, and its effectiveness varies from implantee to implantee.

With these last two points especially in mind, I offer this last anecdote.

* * *

June 2014. Marty and I are on Cumberland, a sea island just off the South Georgia coast. We've taken a ferry across in the morning and hiked through a stunning canopy of live-oak branches, twisted as a cochlea, to the beach on the eastern side, pristine as far as the eye can see. I have a Widex hearing aid in my left ear, my Cochlear Americas processor sitting atop my right. The processor is paired with my ReSound wireless mic, which is hanging from its lanyard around Marty's neck. We stay abreast of each other, walking, talking, and occasionally tossing in an ASL sign.

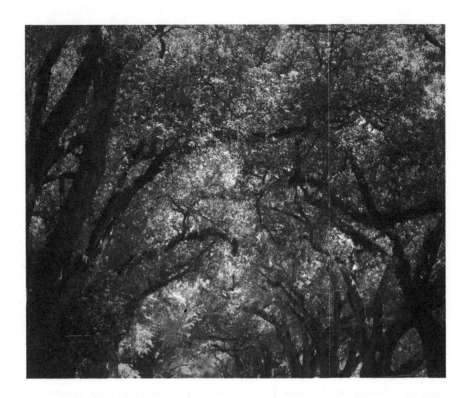

After strolling down the outer beach for a mile and a half, we turn west toward the ferry docks and pass ruins of a Carnegie mansion as big as Downton Abbey. And we begin to see little herds of Cumberland's famed wild horses, though feral or untamed is probably a more accurate term. They look sleek and healthy, like the domestic horses from which they are descended. Some resemble thoroughbreds.

We come upon a particularly gorgeous pair, and Marty circles widely around them hoping to get a better photo, with the early afternoon light behind her. She exceeds the Bluetooth's range, so I turn it off, hoping to hear the horses and the wild turkeys that range free on the island. Spotting some shade, I make my way to a crumbling stone wall about twenty-five yards from her. She's taking pictures with her phone. I pull out our camera, thinking I will snap some neat shots of her snapping the horses.

Suddenly, I hear a rattling sound we're hardwired to fear: Shhsssssssssssss.

I jump forward, doing a silly, hyperkinetic dance like water hitting a hot griddle.

I look for signs of a snake. I see nothing.

I return to my shaded spot and start to photograph Marty and the horses again.

Shhsssssssssssssss!

I jump instinctively again. Now I could be one of the Monty Python players doing a silly walk. I turn and look. Still no snake.

I step back to my shady spot, this time looking straight ahead. I hear the sound again: Shhsssssssssssss.

I look up. Resting on my baseball cap is a dried palmetto frond. With the slightest movement of my head, it scrapes my cap, generating a sound that, to my implant's limited frequency range, sounds like a rattlesnake.

I laugh. After two surgeries, thousands and thousands of dollars, and hours of therapy, I can carry on a pretty decent conversation. But a palmetto frond, encountered for the first time, can still fool me.

I have to laugh. And I have to be grateful.

Snake or no snake, I can hear it.

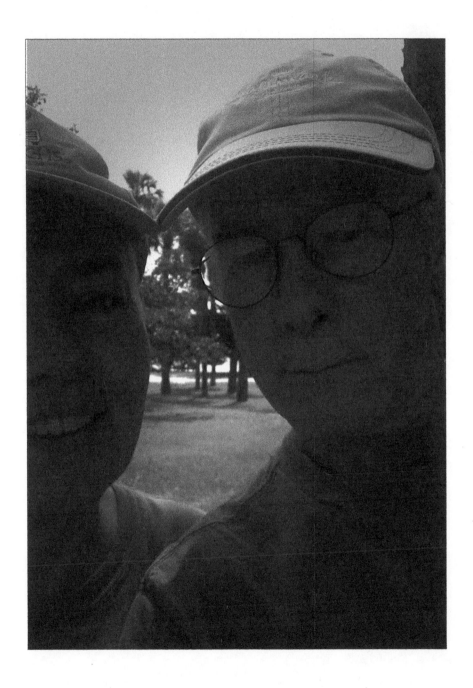

Postscript

Dropping the Needle

I n *The Shawshank Redemption*, the enduringly popular 1998 prison movie based on Stephen King's novella, Andy Dufresne tells his friend and fellow inmate Red how he kept sane while in solitary confinement. He says he had the music of Wolfgang Amadeus Mozart in his head and his heart, safe from the clutches of the warden and the guards.

With music embedded in his memory, imprinted, Andy could drop the needle on the record player in his mind whenever he felt the need. It's a gift, a blessing, that I share. I have come to call it auditory memory. I may be terrible when it comes to remembering faces, but I've always been good with voices. People I hadn't heard from in years would phone me, and quite often I would say, *"Frieda!"* or "Hi, Ronnie," before they had time to identify themselves. Voices just stuck.

Music was much the same. Unlike King's protagonist, I'm not especially tight with Mr. Mozart and his classical cohorts, but I do know a few fugues and arias, some jazz, a smattering of Gilbert and Sullivan, a lot of Rodgers and Hammerstein, and commercial jingles for everything from Ajax "the foaming cleanser" to McCulloch chain saws. I didn't just grow up around music, I was steeped in it. My family sang hymns on Sunday and at Wednesday night prayer meetings. Elementary schools still had music education for kids back then, so we kids at Pendorff Elementary were herded twice a week to the auditorium, where Miss Athalee Poole would lead us through "Hand Me Down My Walking Cane," "Oh! Susanna," and "Sweet Betsy from Pike." My mom, Lucile, and her sister, Nell, had dozens of old 78, everything from Vaughn Monroe to the Andrews Sisters, from Artie Shaw's big band to Spike Jones's screwball combos.

My folks listened to the *Grand Ole Opry* on radio, counted down the Top Ten every week with Snooky Lanson and Gisele MacKenzie on *Your Hit Parade*, and sang along with Mitch Miller, following the bouncing ball through the lyrics to "Heart of My Heart" and "I'm Looking Over a Four-Leaf Clover." I started buying 45s and EPs when I was seven or eight years old—Disney theme songs like "Zorro" and novelty tunes like Sheb Wooley's "Purple People Eater"—and my little brother and I played them over and over and over. We wore the grooves out, as the saying went. Later, I did the same with Elvis Presley's post-Army singles, the Shirelles, Chubby Checker, and Gene Pitney. And when the Beatles conjured up a pantheistic pop-music renaissance, I began to absorb entire albums, not just the mop tops' *Rubber Soul* and *Abbey Road,* but LPs by The Doors, The Who, The Kinks, Otis Redding, Joni Mitchell, Jimi Hendrix, and Carole King.

It's likely that I know at least a verse and the chorus of over five thousand songs, from "Ahab the Arab" to "Zip-a-Dee-Doo-Dah." I didn't consciously commit all these songs and records to memory. It just happened. Call it osmosis. Call it sleep learning. I drifted off to slumber with an LP on the turntable. John Lennon announced that he was the Walrus. I was the Jukebox.

Only a few weeks before my hearing crashed, I started working on a performance piece about this phenomenon. It was part memory poem, part song sampler; and at the time I was writing it, when I not only had hearing but also decent pitch, I could sing each title in tune, running them together into a sort of aural quilt.

I am an old Victrola in my grandmother's parlor

And a cabinet full of scratchy seventy-eights:
Benny Goodman & Doris Day, the Mills Brothers & Danny Kaye
I am a little transistor radio shaped like a rocket ship
I am a tan & white portable phonograph with a fat round spindle
for forty-fives
I am a frayed blue Methodist hymnal at a Wednesday night sing
I am the blinking Wurlitzer jukebox at the Choo Choo Grill
Full up with Marty Robbins and Jackie Wilson
Sam the Sham and Brenda Lee
I am the stereo with fat JBL speakers that helped me and The Who
to rattle a dormitory
"I Can See for Miles" 'cause
"I'm a Believer" and "I Got You Babe," "Baby Lets Play House of
the Rising Sun," son, "Sunday Will Never Be the Same"
"Listen, People":
I have been to "Funkytown" and "St. James Infirmary"
I have been "Sittin' on Top of the World" and "Down in the Valley"
"I Had Too Much to Dream Last Night"
But "That's All Right Mama"
'Cause I am still
That old Victrola at my grandma's house
I'm that rocket-ship radio
I'm that boxy portable phonograph and a pile of forty-fives
I'm that frayed blue hymnal (please turn to Number Sixty-Eight,
"The Old Rugged Cross")
I'm that throbbing, grinning jukebox at the Choo Choo Grill
Full up with truck-driver songs and Roy Orbison operas
Skeeter Davis keening about "The End of the World," Van Morrison
buzzing 'bout his "Brown Eyed Girl"
I'm that stereo system with the big-ass speakers that rattled a dorm
I am CDs of Muddy Waters and Alison Krauss, Marty Winkler
and Steely Dan

And when I go deaf—and I am doing just that—I will still hear it all
Nothing that went in one ear came out the other
I will still hear it all

Acknowledgments

Many friends, family members, journalistic colleagues, and medical professionals helped to make this book a reality, providing everything from moral support to astute suggestions about the manuscript to simply putting up with me and my hearing disability.

I thank Andrew Harris Salomon, Horace Newcomb, Cindy Gary, John Habich, John Huey, Kathleen Ryan, Tim Holston, Ann Holston, Angela Catherine Winkler, Amy Winkler, Mary Padgelek, Michael C. and Melissa Steele, Robin Hardin, Kelly Claas, Dr. Ronald Leif Steenerson, Dr. Karen Hoffmann, Dr. William Slattery, Dr. Dawna Mills, Dr. Eric Robach, David Bianculli, Downie Winkler, Clair Etzold, Xan Holston, Zinnia Larsen Holston, Cam Swiger, Damon Holston and Alice Kirchhoff, Nell Damon, Madeline Van Dyke, Mary Whitehead, Michael Chorost, and Lee Leslie.

Special thanks to Eric Myers, my agent, who got what I was attempting to say, thought it was valuable, and found my publisher, Skyhorse.

Appendix

The US Food and Drug Administration's website—www.fda.gov—has pages devoted to the benefits and risks of various medical devices, including cochlear implants. I did not know this until long after my second surgery. The risk portion is especially telling, covering among other things the loss of taste that I experienced for a while after my first surgery. It would not have made me choose not to have surgery, but it would have been good to know. The FDA speaks to the issue of objective information I mentioned earlier. The agency encourages information seekers to consult its website for updates.

Here's the full FDA list, reprinted with permission from the FDA:

WHAT ARE THE BENEFITS OF COCHLEAR IMPLANT?

- Hearing ranges from near-normal ability to understand speech to *no hearing benefit at all* (italics mine).
- Adults often benefit immediately and continue to improve for about 3 months after the initial tuning sessions. Then, although performance continues to improve, improvements are slower. Cochlear implant users' performances may continue to improve for several years.

- Children may improve at a slower pace. A lot of training is needed after implantation to help the child use the new "hearing" he or she now experiences.
- Most perceive loud, medium and soft sounds. People report that they can perceive different types of sounds, such as footsteps, slamming of doors, sounds of engines, ringing of the telephone, barking of dogs, whistling of the tea kettle, rustling of leaves, the sound of a light switch being switched on and off, and so on.
- Many understand speech without lip-reading. However, even if this is not possible, using the implant helps lip-reading.
- Many can make telephone calls and understand familiar voices over the telephone. Some good performers can make normal telephone calls and even understand an unfamiliar speaker. However, not all people who have implants are able to use the phone.
- Many can watch TV more easily, especially when they can also see the speaker's face. However, listening to the radio is often more difficult as there are no visual cues available.
- Some can enjoy music. Some enjoy the sound of certain instruments (piano or guitar, for example) and certain voices. Others do not hear well enough to enjoy music

WHAT ARE THE RISKS OF COCHLEAR IMPLANTS?

GENERAL ANESTHESIA RISKS

- General anesthesia is drug-induced sleep. The drugs, such as anesthetic gases and injected drugs, may affect people differently. For most people, the risk of general anesthesia is very low. However, for some people with certain medical conditions, it is more risky.

RISKS FROM THE SURGICAL IMPLANT PROCEDURE

- Injury to the facial nerve—this nerve goes through the middle ear to give movement to the muscles of the face. It lies close to where the surgeon needs to place the implant, and thus it can be injured during the surgery. An injury can cause a temporary or permanent weakening or full paralysis on the same side of the face as the implant.
- Meningitis—this is an infection of the lining of the surface of the brain. People who have abnormally formed inner ear structures appear to be at greater risk of this rare, but serious complication. For more information on the risk of meningitis in cochlear recipients, see the nearby Useful Links.
- Cerebrospinal fluid leakage—the brain is surrounded by fluid that may leak from a hole created in the inner ear or elsewhere from a hole in the covering of the brain as a result of the surgical procedure.
- Perilymph fluid leak—the inner ear or cochlea contains fluid. This fluid can leak through the hole that was created to place the implant.
- Infection of the skin wound.
- Blood or fluid collection at the site of surgery.
- Attacks of dizziness or vertigo.
- Tinnitus, which is a ringing or buzzing sound in the ear.
- Taste disturbances—the nerve that gives taste sensation to the tongue also goes through the middle ear and might be injured during the surgery.
- Numbness around the ear.
- Reparative granuloma—this is the result of localized inflammation that can occur if the body rejects the implant.
- There may be other unforeseen complications that could occur with long term implantation that we cannot now predict.

OTHER RISKS ASSOCIATED WITH THE USE OF COCHLEAR IMPLANTS

PEOPLE WITH A COCHLEAR IMPLANT:

- May hear sounds differently. Sound impressions from an implant differ from normal hearing, according to people who could hear before they became deaf. At first, users describe the sound as "mechanical," "technical," or "synthetic." This perception changes over time, and most users do not notice this artificial sound quality after a few weeks of cochlear implant use.
- May lose residual hearing. The implant may destroy any remaining hearing in the implanted ear.
- May have unknown and uncertain effects. The cochlear implant stimulates the nerves directly with electrical currents. Although this stimulation appears to be safe, the long-term effect of these electrical currents on the nerves is unknown.
- May not hear as well as others who have had successful outcomes with their implants.
- May not be able to understand language well. There is no test a person can take before surgery that will predict how well he or she will understand language after surgery.
- May have to have it removed temporarily or permanently if an infection develops after the implant surgery. However, this is a rare complication.
- May have their implant fail. In this situation, a person with an implant would need to have additional surgery to resolve this problem and would be exposed to the risks of surgery again.
- May not be able to upgrade their implant when new external components become available. Implanted parts are usually compatible with improved external parts. That way, as

advances in technology develop, one can upgrade his or her implant by changing only its external parts. In some cases, though, this won't work and the implant will need changing.

- May not be able to have some medical examinations and treatments. These treatments include:
  - ○ MRI imaging. MRI is becoming a more routine diagnostic method for early detection of medical problems. Even being close to an MRI imaging unit will be dangerous because it may dislodge the implant or demagnetize its internal magnet. FDA has approved some implants, however, for some types of MRI studies done under controlled conditions.
  - ○ neurostimulation.
  - ○ electrical surgery.
  - ○ electroconvulsive therapy.
  - ○ ionic radiation therapy.
- Will depend on batteries for hearing. For some devices new or recharged batteries are needed every day.
- May damage their implant. Contact sports, automobile accidents, slips and falls, or other impacts near the ear can damage the implant. This may mean needing a new implant and more surgery. It is unknown whether a new implant would work as well as the old one.
- May find them expensive. Replacing damaged or lost parts may be expensive.
- Will have to use it for the rest of life. During a person's lifetime, the manufacturer of the cochlear implant could go out of business. Whether a person will be able to get replacement parts or other customer service in the future is uncertain.
- May have lifestyle changes because their implant will interact with the electronic environment. An implant may
  - ○ set off theft detection systems.
  - ○ set off metal detectors or other security systems.

        ○   be affected by cellular phone users or other radio transmitters.

        ○   have to be turned off during takeoffs and landings in aircraft.

        ○   interact in unpredictable ways with other computer systems.

- Will have to be careful of static electricity. Static electricity may temporarily or permanently damage a cochlear implant. It may be good practice to remove the processor and headset before contact with static generating materials such as children's plastic play equipment, TV screens, computer monitors, or synthetic fabric. For more details regarding how to deal with static electricity, contact the manufacturer or implant center.

- Have less ability to hear both soft sounds and loud sounds without changing the sensitivity of the implant. The sensitivity of normal hearing is adjusted continuously by the brain, but the design of cochlear implants requires that a person manually change sensitivity setting of the device as the sound environment changes.

- May develop irritation where the external part rubs on the skin and have to remove it for a while.

- Can't let the external parts get wet. Damage from water may be expensive to repair and the person may be without hearing until the implant is repaired. Thus, the person will need to remove the external parts of the device when bathing, showering, swimming, or participating in water sports.

- May hear strange sounds caused by its interaction with magnetic fields, like those near airport passenger screening machines.

Song Credits

Paul McCartney, "Tug of War," © Kobalt Music Publishing Ltd.

Paul McCartney, John Lennon, "Eleanor Rigby," © Sony/ATV Music Publishing LLC

Billy Hayes, Jay W. Johnson, "Blue Christmas," © Universal Music Publishing Group, Demi Music Corp., D/B/A Lichelle Music Company

Ross Bagdasarian Sr., "Witch Doctor," © Sony/ATV Music Publishing LLC

Jerome J. Garcia, Philip Lesh, Robert C. Hunter, Robert Hall Weir, "Truckin'," © Universal Music Publishing Group

SONGS EVOKED BY TITLE IN THE POSTSCRIPT

Peter Townsend, "I Can See for Miles," © T.R.O. Inc.

Neil Diamond, "I'm a Believer," © Sony/ATV Music Publishing LLC, Universal Music Publishing Group.

Sonny Bono, "I Got You, Babe," © Warner/Chappell Music, Inc.

Arthur Gunter, "Baby Let's Play House," © Music Sales Corporation, BMG Rights Management.

"House of the Rising Sun," traditional.

Terry Cashman, Gene Pistilli, "Sunday Will Never Be the Same," © Universal Music Publishing Group.

Ernestine Madison, Frank Wilson, Frank Edward Wilson, "Listen

People," © Sony/ATV Music Publishing LLC, Warner/Chappell Music, Inc.

Steve Greenberg, "Funkytown," © Warner/Chappell Music, Inc.

Joe Primrose, Irving Mills, "St. James Infirmary," © Sony/ATV Music Publishing LLC, Universal Music Publishing Group, Downtown Music Publishing, Spirit Music Group, BMG Rights Management.

Walter Vinson, Lonnie Chatmon, "Sittin' on Top of the World," © Warner Chappell Music, Inc.

Solomon Burke, Marvin Chivian, Joseph C. Martin, Bert Berns, "Down in the Valley," © Warner Chappell Music, Inc, Kobalt Music Publishing Ltd.

Annette Tucker, Nancie Mantz, "I Had Too Much to Dream Last Night," © Sony/ATV Music Publishing LLC.

Arthur Crudup, "That's All Right Mama," © Warner Chappell Music, Inc.

George Bennard, "The Old Rugged Cross,"© Warner Chappell Music, Inc.

Peter Mcnulty-Connolly, Marcus Mybe, Louie St. Louis, Kurtis Deshaun Williams, Michael Angelo, "The End Of The World," © Universal Music Publishing Group, Sony/ATV Music Publishing LLC.

Van Morrison, "Brown Eyed Girl," © Universal Music Publishing Group.